Illustrated Pathology of the Bone Marrow

This book provides a highly illustrated overview of the diseases of the human bone marrow. It will help experienced clinicians and those in training to answer the practical diagnostic questions that arise during the routine analysis of bone marrow core biopsy specimens. Throughout the text, histologic interpretation is integrated with clinical and laboratory findings. Emphasis is placed on the evaluation of peripheral blood, aspirate smear, clot section, and core biopsy, as well as ancillary techniques including flow cytometry and immunohistochemistry, in the diagnosis of hematologic disorders of the marrow. The text is illustrated with numerous color figures, charts, and tables, and descriptions of real case situations using the most up-to-date classification systems. *Illustrated Pathology of the Bone Marrow* should be read by all pathologists, hematologists, and laboratory technicians involved in the analysis of bone marrow specimens.

Attilio Orazi is Professor of Pathology and Director of the Division of Hematopathology at Indiana University School of Medicine.

Dennis O'Malley is Assistant Professor in the Division of Hematopathology at Indiana University School of Medicine.

Daniel Arber is Professor of Pathology and Associate Chair of Pathology for Hematopathology at Stanford University Medical Center.

Illustrated Pathology of the Bone Marrow

Attilio Orazi

Indiana University School of Medicine

Dennis P. O'Malley

Indiana University School of Medicine

Daniel A. Arber

Stanford University Medical Center

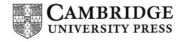

CAMBRIDGE UNIVERSITY PRESS
Cambridge, New York, Melbourne, Madrid, Cape Town, Singapore, São Paulo

Cambridge University Press
The Edinburgh Building, Cambridge CB2 8RU, UK

Published in the United States of America by Cambridge University Press, New York

www.cambridge.org
Information on this title: www.cambridge.org/9780521810036

First published 2006
Reprinted 2007

Printed in the United Kingdom at the University Press, Cambridge

A catalog record for this publication is available from the British Library

Library of Congress Cataloging in Publication data
Orazi, Attilio.
Illustrated pathology of the bone marrow/Attilio Orazi, Dennis P.
O'Malley, Daniel A. Arber.
    p. cm.
Includes bibliographical references and index.
ISBN-13: 978-0-521-81003-6 (hardback)
ISBN-10: 0-521-81003-5 (hardback)
1. Bone marrow – Diseases – Atlases. I. O'Malley, Dennis P., 1965– II. Arber, Daniel A., 1961– III. Title.
[DNLM: 1. Bone Marrow – pathology. 2. Bone marrow Cells – pathology. 3. Bone Marrow Neoplasms/diagnosis.
4. Cell Proliferation. WH 380 063i 2006]
RC645.7073 2006
616.4′107 – dc22   2006010121

ISBN-13 978-0-521-81003-6 hardback

To my parents, to Maria, my wife and best friend, and to Giulia and Rita, our marvelous daughters – AO

To my wife, Karene, who is always there to support me – DPO

To my parents and to my wife, Carol – DAA

Contents

Preface

Illustrated Pathology of the Bone Marrow is designed to help pathologists and pathologists in training answer the practical diagnostic questions that arise during routine analysis of bone marrow core biopsy specimens. Although emphasis has been placed on the histologic interpretation of the bone marrow biopsy, an attempt has been made to integrate histologic findings with clinical and laboratory features and peripheral blood and bone marrow aspiration morphology. In recent years, integration between morphology, immunophenotype, genetic features, and clinical features has been increasingly used to distinguish between distinct clinical entities. This integrated multiparametric approach forms the basis for the WHO classification of tumors of hematopoietic and lymphoid tissue. As a consequence, morphology, immunophenotype, genetics, and clinical features are integrated throughout the book in an effort to summarize the current best practice of bone marrow interpretation. The illustrative case material in this book has been gathered from several institutions, including Indiana University School of Medicine in Indianapolis, Indiana; the College of Physicians and Surgeons of Columbia University, New York, New York; the City of Hope National Medical Center, Duarte, California; and Stanford University, Stanford, California. A systematic, analytical approach to interpretation of pathological changes is used throughout the book, which will enable pathologists with varying backgrounds and experience to feel confident in their assessment of bone marrow specimens during their routine everyday analysis.

Each of us owes a great debt to those who taught us and influenced us. We have each learned a great deal from "giants" in the field of pathology and we wish to acknowledge at least some of those who had the greatest impact on us: Franco Rilke, Richard S. Neiman, Peter M. Banks, Thomas F. Dutcher, Henry Rappaport, and Lawrence M. Weiss.

We would like to thank our colleagues, trainees and technical staff who contributed to the production of this book. We would like to thank the following for providing case materials for use in this book: Caroline An, Peter Banks, Magdalena Czader, Milton Drachenberg, Anselm Hii, Steve Kroft, Stephen Lee, Irma Pereira, Sherrie Perkins, Jonathon Perry, Kenneth Ryder, Jess Savala, Saeed Vakili, Gail Vance, Patrick Ward, and the Indiana University Cytogenetics Laboratory.

Special thanks to Regina Bennett for her excellent technical assistance.

Introduction

Indications for bone marrow examination

Bone marrow examination, including both aspiration and biopsy sampling, can be performed on virtually any patient. However, patients with coagulation deficiencies or profound thrombocytopenia may experience prolonged bleeding, which cannot be controlled by pressure bandages. In these rare cases, specific treatment (e.g., platelet transfusion) may be indicated. Indications for performing bone marrow examination are summarized in Table 1.1. In the vast majority of cases, both a bone marrow aspiration and biopsy should be performed. Bone marrow aspiration and bone marrow biopsy are complementary (Bain, 2001a, 2001b). Bone marrow aspiration provides excellent cytologic detail; however, marrow architecture cannot be assessed. Bone marrow core biopsy allows for an accurate analysis of architecture; however, cytologic details may be lost. Table 1.2 shows the accepted indications for performing a bone marrow biopsy. This includes cases with inadequate or failed aspiration, need for accurate assessment of cellularity, cases in which the presence of focal lesions (e.g., granulomatous disease or metastatic carcinoma) is suspected, suspected bone marrow fibrosis, need to study bone marrow architecture, need to study bone structure, bone marrow stroma, or assessment of bone marrow vascularity. In general, patients with hypocellular marrows or bone marrow fibrosis are likely to need a trephine biopsy for adequate assessment. In such patients, an aspirate would probably be inadequate or even impossible. Unexplained pancytopenia and unexplained leukoerythroblastic blood pictures are further indications for a biopsy, because they are likely to indicate the presence of bone marrow metastatic disease or fibrosis.

The bone marrow biopsy specimen differs from biopsy material from most other organs, because a proper interpretation of the bone marrow requires the incorporation of a variety of specimen types and often ancillary techniques to arrive at an accurate and complete diagnosis. Bone marrow studies should be evaluated in conjunction with clinical data, peripheral blood smears, and complete blood count data as well as with bone marrow aspirate smears or imprints. Occasionally, bone marrow biopsy imprint smears may be used to assess cytology in cases with inaspirable marrows (dry taps). Many cases also benefit from cytochemical evaluation of marrow aspirate smears, flow cytometric immunophenotyping, immunohistochemical staining of bone marrow biopsy, molecular genetic and cytogenetic studies. The results of all of these should be considered in making a final diagnosis. The following chapters will emphasize this multi-factorial approach to bone marrow evaluation and attempt to highlight the diagnostic questions that require the use of ancillary techniques for accurate diagnosis. Complete clinical information is also necessary for the proper triage of the types of samples/tests required to provide the most comprehensive diagnostic information.

Obtaining the bone marrow biopsy

The technique used to obtain bone marrow aspirate smears has been described in detail previously, and the reader is referred to those publications for more detail (Brynes *et al.*, 1978; Brunning & McKenna, 1994; Perkins, 1999; Foucar, 2001). If bone marrow aspiration and bone marrow biopsy are both being performed using the same needle, it is usually preferable to obtain the biopsy first, to avoid distortion of the biopsy specimen by aspiration artifacts. Another approach uses separate needles for each procedure. This requires that the needles be placed in different sites of the bone marrow; good-quality aspirate and biopsy can be obtained in either sequence. When two needles are used,

Table 1.1. Indications for a bone marrow aspiration with or without a trephine biopsy.

Investigation and/or follow-up of

Unexplained microcytosis
Unexplained macrocytosis
Unexplained anemia
Unexplained thrombocytopenia
Pancytopenia (including suspected aplastic anemia)
Leukoerythroblastic blood smear and suspected bone marrow infiltration
Suspected acute leukemia
Assessment of remission status after treatment of acute leukemia
Suspected myelodysplastic syndrome or myelodysplastic/myeloproliferative disorder
Suspected chronic myeloproliferative disorder (chronic myelogenous leukemia, polycythemia rubra vera, essential thrombocythemia, idiopathic myelofibrosis, or systemic mastocytosis)
Suspected chronic lymphocytic leukemia and other leukemic lymphoproliferative disorders
Suspected non-Hodgkin lymphoma
Suspected hairy cell leukemia
Staging of non-Hodgkin lymphoma
Suspected multiple myeloma or other plasma cell dyscrasia
Suspected storage disease
Fever of unknown origin
Confirmation of normal bone marrow if bone marrow is being aspirated for allogeneic transplantation

Table 1.2. Indications for performing a bone marrow biopsy.

Investigation and/or follow-up of

Diagnosis and/or staging of suspected Hodgkin lymphoma and non-Hodgkin lymphoma
Hairy cell leukemia
Chronic lymphocytic leukemia and other leukemic lymphoproliferative disorders
Diagnosis of suspected metastatic carcinoma
Diagnosis, staging, and follow-up of small cell tumors of childhood
Chronic myeloproliferative disorders (chronic myelogenous leukemia, polycythaemia rubra vera, essential thrombocythemia, idiopathic myelofibrosis, and mastocytosis)
Diagnosis of aplastic anemia
Investigation of an unexplained leukoerythroblastic blood smear
Investigation of a fever of unknown origin and/or granulomatous infection
Investigation of suspected hemophagocytic syndrome
Evaluation of any patient in whom an adequate bone marrow aspirate cannot be obtained
Suspected multiple myeloma or plasma cell dyscrasia
Suspected acute myeloid leukemia
Suspected myelodysplastic syndrome
Investigation of suspected storage disease
Suspected primary amyloidosis
Investigation of bone diseases

it is often advantageous to aspirate the marrow through a smaller needle specifically designed for that purpose. This minimizes the contamination with peripheral blood, which is often observed when the aspirate is performed through the Jamshidi needle. The skin and periosteum are infiltrated with 1% xylocaine. The bone marrow aspiration needle is introduced into the medullary cavity as for bone marrow biopsy. Once the medullary cavity has been entered, the stylus is removed and a syringe attached. The marrow is aspirated by rapidly pulling back on the syringe. Optimally, this should last less than five seconds and yields not more than 1 milliliter of bone marrow aspirate material. Any additional material which can be aspirated will be mostly peripheral blood.

The initial aspirate sample should always be used for morphology. Subsequent aspirations may be obtained for flow cytometry, cytogenetics, microbiology culture, or molecular studies. Non-anticoagulated specimens should be immediately handed to a technical assistant who will prepare various smears and bone marrow particle crush preparations. The remaining marrow aspirate material is allowed to clot and submitted for marrow clot sections.

Alternatively, aspirate smears can be made in the laboratory after the procedure. To this end, bone marrow aspirate material should be immediately placed into tubes (generally coded with purple tops in the USA) containing ethylenediaminetetraacetic acid (EDTA). This metal limits the clotting of the aspirate specimen and allows material to be submitted for ancillary studies as well as particle sections. Whether the smears are made at the bedside or from the EDTA tubes, the aspirate should be grossly evaluated for the presence of bone marrow particles. The absence of particles on a smear limits its diagnostic usefulness in many cases. Such smears often show findings consistent with peripheral blood contamination. Many pediatric patients, however, will not demonstrate gross particles in the aspirate material despite numerous bone marrow elements in the smear.

Representative aspirate smears and imprints are stained with a Romanovsky type of stain. The actual stain type varies among laboratories and includes Giemsa, Wright–Giemsa, and May–Grunwald–Giemsa stains. We prefer the Wright–Giemsa stain. Rapid review of these smears helps in determining the need for ancillary studies, such as cytochemistry, immunophenotyping, cytogenetic analysis, and molecular genetic study.

Clot biopsy sections are often made from coagulated aspirate material. This material contains predominantly blood as well as small marrow particles that can be embedded in paraffin, sectioned, and stained with hematoxylin and eosin (H&E) or other stains. Alternatively, when EDTA-anticoagulated aspirate specimens are used, the bone marrow particles that are left after smears are prepared can be filtered and embedded for histologic evaluation (Arber *et al.*, 1993). This method provides a more concentrated collection of marrow particles but may not yield any material, particularly in pediatric patients (Brunning *et al.*, 1975).

Trephine core biopsy is not performed for all patients, but these specimens are essential in the evaluation of patients suspected of having disease that may only focally involve the bone marrow, such as malignant lymphoma or metastatic carcinoma, and are preferred in all patients. Core biopsies allow for architectural assessment of the bone marrow and offer a number of other benefits. The incidences of bone marrow involvement by various types of malignancies are proportional to the amount of bone marrow evaluated. Review of the published findings suggests that the minimum adequate length is in the range 15 to 20 mm. One study of the relation between length of trephine and the rate of positivity for neoplasia yielded a minimum adequate length of 12 mm in section (16 mm before processing; trephine biopsies shrank by 25% during processing). The authors reported that 58% of the trephines performed in their institution were inadequate by this criterion (Bishop *et al.*, 1992). To increase the yield, bilateral bone marrow biopsies have been recommended for patients undergoing bone marrow staging by several authors (Brunning *et al.*, 1975; Wang *et al.*, 2002). The adequacy of a random iliac crest biopsy marrow sampling for detection of metastatic malignancy is, however, still controversial. Recent results have suggested that, if the diagnosis of bone marrow isolated tumor cells has clinical relevance, the preoperative assessment should be performed by rib segment resection or methods other than iliac crest aspirate and/or biopsy (Mattioli *et al.*, 2001). Further investigation is needed to determine whether isolated tumor cells have a preferential spread to bones other than the ileum.

Imprint slides from the biopsy specimens may yield positive same-day results in some of the aspirate-negative or dry-tap cases (James *et al.*, 1980). The imprints can be made either at the bedside or in the laboratory. To make them in the laboratory, the bone marrow core is submitted fresh, on saline-dampened gauze, with the imprints made immediately to allow adequate fixation of the biopsy specimen.

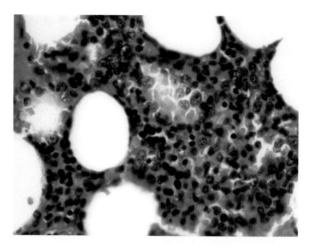

Figure 1.1. An example of a poorly prepared bone marrow core biopsy. The specimen is too thick and not well stained, preventing adequate identification of different cell types and their stages of maturation.

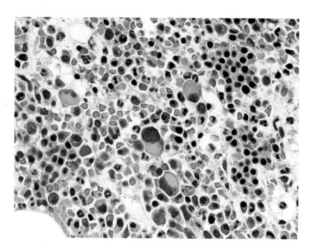

Figure 1.2. An example of a well-sectioned and well-stained core biopsy. Thin sections and a well-performed H&E stain of the core biopsy section are imperative for adequate interpretation.

Otherwise, the imprints are made at the bedside, and the biopsy specimen is submitted in fixative.

Many laboratories prefer mercuric chloride-based fixatives (e.g., B5) or Bouin's fixative for bone marrow specimens. Submission of the bone marrow biopsy material in formalin followed by EDTA or short nitric acid decalcification also provides more than acceptable results. After fixation and decalcification, the core biopsy specimen is stained with H&E and other stains. The need for well-prepared thin bone marrow biopsy sections cannot be overemphasized. Thick, poorly processed specimens (Fig. 1.1) are almost useless. A properly processed section stained with H&E is shown in Fig. 1.2.

REFERENCES

Arber, D. A., Johnson, R. M., Rainer, P. A., Helbert, B., Chang, K. L., & Rappaport, E. S. (1993). The bone marrow agar section: a morphologic and immunohistochemical evaluation. *Modern Pathology*, **6**, 592–8.

Bain, B. J. (2001a). Bone marrow aspiration. *Journal of Clinical Pathology*, **54**, 657–63.

Bain, B. J. (2001b). Bone marrow trephine biopsy. *Journal of Clinical Pathology*, **54**, 737–42.

Bishop, P. W., McNally, K., & Harris, M. (1992). Audit of bone marrow trephines. *Journal of Clinical Pathology*, **45**, 1105–8.

Brunning, R. D. & McKenna, R. W. (1994). Appendix: bone marrow specimen processing. In *Tumors of the Bone Marrow: Atlas of Tumor Pathology*. Third Series, Fascicle 9. Washington, DC: Armed Forces Institute of Pathology, pp. 475–89.

Brunning, R. D., Bloomfield, C. D., McKenna, R. W., & Peterson, L. A. (1975). Bilateral trephine bone marrow biopsies in lymphoma and other neoplastic diseases. *Annals of Internal Medicine*, **82**, 365–6.

Brynes, R. K., McKenna, R. W., & Sundberg R. D. (1978). Bone marrow aspiration and trephine biopsy: an approach to a thorough study. *American Journal of Clinical Pathology*, **70**, 753–9.

Foucar, K. (2001). Bone marrow examination techniques. In *Bone Marrow Pathology*, 2nd edn. Chicago, IL: ASCP Press, pp. 30–47.

James, L. P., Stass, S. A., & Schumacher, H. R. (1980). Value of imprint preparations of bone marrow biopsies in hematologic diagnosis. *Cancer*, **46**, 173–7.

Mattioli, S., D'Ovidio, F., Tazzari, P., *et al.* (2001). Iliac crest biopsy versus rib segment resection for the detection of bone marrow isolated tumor cells from lung and esophageal cancer. *European Journal of Cardiothoracic Surgery*, **19**, 576–9.

Perkins, S. L. (1999). Examination of the blood and bone marrow. In *Wintrobe's Clinical Hematology*, 10th edn., ed. G. R. Lee, J. Foerster, J. Lukens, *et al.* Baltimore, MD: Williams & Wilkins, pp. 9–35.

Wang, J., Weiss, L. M., Chang, K. L., *et al.* (2002). Diagnostic utility of bilateral bone marrow examination: significance of morphologic and ancillary technique study in malignancy. *Cancer*, **94**, 1522–31.

The normal bone marrow and an approach to bone marrow evaluation of neoplastic and proliferative processes

Introduction

It is often easiest to evaluate a bone marrow specimen by comparing it to what would be expected in the normal bone marrow (Brown & Gatter, 1993; Bain, 1996). The initial evaluation on low magnification includes the assessment of sample adequacy and marrow cellularity. The latter is usually based on the biopsy. Estimates of cellularity on aspirate material have been described (Fong, 1979) but may be unreliable in variably cellular marrows (Gruppo et al., 1997). The normal cellularity varies with age (Table 2.1), and evaluation of cellularity must always be made in the context of the patient's age (Hartsock et al., 1965) (Fig. 2.1). The marrow is approximately 100% cellular during the first three months of life, 80% cellular in children through age 10 years; it then slowly declines in cellularity until age 30 years, when it remains about 50% cellular. The usually accepted range of cellularity in normal adults is 40–70% (Hartsock et al., 1965; Gulati et al., 1988; Bain, 1996; Friebert et al., 1998; Naeim, 1998). The marrow cellularity declines again in elderly patients to about 30% at 70 years. Because of the variation in cellularity by age, the report should clearly indicate whether the stated cellularity in a given specimen is normocellular, hypocellular, or hypercellular.

Estimates of cellularity may be inappropriately lowered by several factors. Subcortical bone marrow is normally hypocellular, and the first three subcortical trabecular spaces are usually ignored in the cellularity estimate (Fig. 2.2). Superficial core biopsies may contain only these subcortical areas, and such biopsy specimens should be considered inadequate for purpose of cellularity evaluation. Technical artifacts may also falsely lower marrow cellularity. Tears made in the section during processing and cutting as well as artifactual displacement of marrow from bony trabeculae should not be considered in the estimate. Likewise, crush artifact may falsely elevate the cellularity.

After the marrow cellularity has been evaluated, the cellular elements must be considered (Table 2.2). The three main bone marrow cell lineages, erythroid, myeloid (granulocytic), and megakaryocytic, should be evaluated first. Maturing myeloid cells are the most common cell type in normal marrow, with a 2 : 1 to 4 : 1 myeloid-to-erythroid (M : E) ratio; the higher ratio is more common in women and young children. All stages of granulocyte and erythroid maturation are normally present, with blast cells usually less than 3%. The various stages of cell maturation are best evaluated from the aspirate smear material, but the distribution pattern of different cell lineages is best evaluated on the clot or core biopsy specimen (Frisch & Bartl, 1999) (Fig. 2.3). Granulopoietic precursors normally occur adjacent to bone trabeculae. Erythroblasts and megakaryocytes are predominantly found in the central regions of the marrow cavities, often adjacent to sinusoids. Erythroblasts are found in small and large clusters of cells exhibiting the full range of maturational stages from the proerythroblasts to the orthrochromatic normoblasts. Megakaryocytes are easily identifiable on smear and biopsy material in the normal marrow and should consist of predominantly mature forms (>15 μm diameter) with multilobated nuclei.

Lymphocytes normally represent 10% to 15% of cells on aspirate smears, but lymphoid precursor cells (hematogones) and mature lymphocytes may be normally increased in children and the elderly, respectively. Lymphoid precursors (Longacre et al., 1989) are less obvious in the biopsy material of children, despite being evident on aspirate smears. Lymphoid aggregates are common in biopsy material of elderly patients and are non-paratrabecular in location (Fig. 2.4). The aggregates are more commonly predominantly composed of T lymphocytes. Cells that are present at a lower frequency in the bone marrow include monocytes, plasma cells,

Table 2.1. Age-related normal values in bone marrow.

Age	% Cellularity	% Granulocyte	% Erythroid	% Lymphocytes
Newborn	80–100	50	40	10
1–3 months	80–100	50–60	5–10	30–50
Child	60–80	50–60	20	20–30
Adult	40–70	50–70	20–25	10–15

Adapted from Foucar, 2001

Table 2.2. Normal adult values for bone marrow differential cell counts.

Cell type	Normal range (%)
Myeloblasts	0–3
Promyelocytes	2–8
Myelocytes	10–13
Metamyelocytes	10–15
Band/neutrophils	25–40
Eosinophils and precursors	1–3
Basophils and precursors	0–1
Monocytes	0–1
Erythroblasts	0–2
Other erythroid elements	15–25
Lymphocytes	10–15
Plasma cells	0–1

Adapted from Foucar, 2001

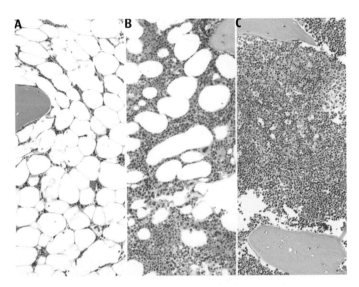

Figure 2.1. Examples of the ranges of cellularity seen in bone marrow: (A) a markedly hypocellular bone marrow (<5% cellularity), (B) approximately 40% cellularity, and (C) bone marrow with nearly 100% cellularity.

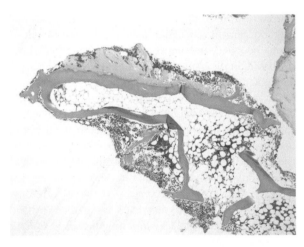

Figure 2.2. An example of a core biopsy taken in a subcortical location. Note the periosteum (upper portion of the photograph), suggesting that this is the outer cortical layer of the bone. Beneath this outer cortex of bone there is an area of hypocellular bone marrow which includes the first three subcortical trabecular spaces. Deeper in the specimen (lower right corner), the cellularity is considered to be more representative.

mast cells, eosinophils, basophils, and osteoblasts. These cells normally represent less than 5% of marrow cells on smears.

Cells and proliferations that do not normally occur in the marrow, including histiocyte accumulations or granulomas, fibrosis, serous atrophy, and neoplastic cells, should be systematically assessed in all specimens. The bone trabeculae should also be evaluated for evidence of osteopenia, osteoblastic proliferations, and changes of Paget's disease (Frisch & Bartl, 1999). However, detailed evaluation of metabolic bone diseases requires special techniques such as undecalcified biopsies embedded in plastic, in vitro tetracycline labeling, and histomorphometry (Teitelbaum & Bullough, 1979). A detailed discussion of bone pathology is beyond the scope of this book, which is primarily devoted to bone marrow interpretation.

Evaluation of stainable iron

Marrow aspirate smears

In a normal bone marrow aspirate smear stained by Prussian blue, iron is predominantly found in histiocytes embedded inside marrow particles (Fig. 2.5). Iron incorporation in erythroid cells is also normally seen in scattered erythroblasts that usually demonstrate one or two siderotic

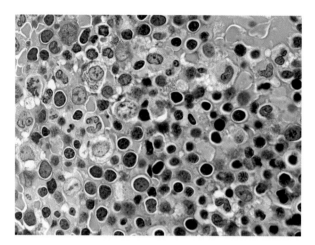

Figure 2.3. Erythroid and myeloid precursors in a clot section. Erythroid precursors typically have perfectly round nuclei with variable amounts of cytoplasm, which may appear clear.

Table 2.3. Grading of iron storage in bone marrow aspirate material.

Grade	Characteristic
0 or negative	No iron identified under oil immersion
1+	Small iron-positive particles visible only under oil immersion
2+	Small, sparsely distributed iron particles usually visible under low magnification
3+	Numerous small particles present in histiocytes throughout the marrow particles
4+	Larger particles throughout the marrow with tendency to aggregate into clumps
5+	Dense, large clumps of iron throughout the marrow
6+	Large deposits of iron, both intracellular and extracellular, that obscure cellular detail in the marrow particles

Adapted from Gale *et al.*, 1963

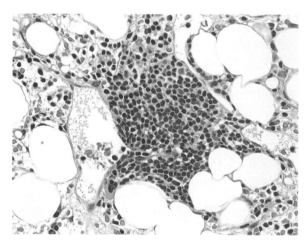

Figure 2.4. A benign lymphoid aggregate within a bone marrow biopsy. This lymphoid aggregate, which is composed predominantly of small lymphocytes, most likely represents a reactive lymphoid follicle. Note that the aggregate is in a perivascular location, which is most often associated with benign lymphoid aggregates.

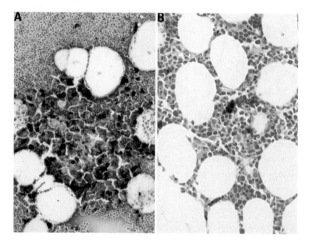

Figure 2.5. Iron stains on bone marrows. (A) An iron stain on an aspirate smear shows a markedly increased amount of stainable iron. (B) Iron staining on a bone marrow core biopsy, which typically under-represents the amount of iron present. This is due to the iron solubilization effect that occurs during histologic tissue processing. The loss can be partially prevented by using non-acid decalcification methods.

granules adjacent to the nucleus (sideroblasts). Grading of marrow iron content is outlined in Table 2.3.

Bone marrow biopsy

Biopsy decalcification removes iron. Decalcified sections, therefore, underestimate iron stores and may give the misleading impression of iron deficiency. Iron stores are more accurately reflected in plastic-embedded sections (undecalcified) and in clot section preparations, if adequate marrow particles are present (Fig. 2.5). Hemosiderin may also

be visible in H&E-stained sections of marrow as coarse golden-brown granules in macrophages. The presence of visible hemosiderin in H&E-stained marrow sections usually indicates increased iron stores (Strauchen, 1996).

Evaluation of bone marrow extracellular stroma, marrow fibrosis, and mesenchymal cells

The extracellular matrix is demonstrable in routine preparations by reticulin (Gomori) silver stain, which stains most

Table 2.4. Grading of bone marrow fibrosis.

1+	Focal fine fibers with only rare coarse fibers
2+	A diffuse fine fiber network with an increase in scattered coarse fibers
3+	A diffuse coarse fiber network with no collagenization (negative trichrome stain)
4+	A diffuse fiber network with collagenization (positive trichrome stain)

Modified from Manoharan *et al.*, 1979

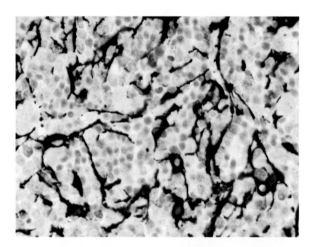

Figure 2.6. An immunohistochemical stain for low-affinity nerve growth factor receptor (LNGFR), highlighting bone marrow adventitial reticular cells (ARC). Note the characteristic dendritic morphology of the ARC.

types of collagen including collagen III and collagen IV, and by collagen IV immunostain, which stains the basal membrane collagen type. Bone marrow reticulum cells, also termed adventitial reticular cells, can be identified by their nerve growth factor receptor positivity (NGFR) (Cattoretti *et al.*, 1993). In most cases, the amount of NGFR staining roughly parallels the degree of reticulin fibrosis (Fig. 2.6).

Evaluation of fibrosis

Assessment for the presence and degree of marrow fibrosis is usually done by staining marrow sections with the Gomori silver stain technique. The degree of fibrosis can be estimated by using the approach proposed by Manoharan *et al.* (1979) (see Table 2.4). Trichrome stain (e.g., Masson's) is commonly used to demonstrate the presence of "mature" collagen, which can occur in advanced stages of marrow fibrosis (i.e., osteomyelosclerosis). The grading of fibrosis, as a general rule, should be performed taking into account only areas of active hematopoiesis (fatty areas are

excluded). In pathological bone marrow, areas of prominent stroma alterations, such as those with marked edema or extensive fibrosclerosis, should also be included in the overall grading of the myelofibrosis.

Ancillary techniques useful in bone marrow evaluation

Ancillary techniques are essential for the proper diagnosis of many bone marrow neoplasms. Because therapy is now often specific for the exact type of the neoplastic cells and prognosis is often directly related to genetic changes associated with various types of neoplasm, the tests described here are often vital for a proper evaluation of the patient. Despite remarkable advances in immunophenotyping and cancer genetics, morphologic evaluation still remains a crucial step in the assessment of the bone marrow. In most cases, morphologic findings guide the pathologist in the selection of appropriate additional studies, to identify clinically significant immunophenotypic and genetic findings. These morphologic features are discussed with the specific diseases, as are the specific findings of the various ancillary tests. The general utility and applications of ancillary testing, however, are discussed here.

Cytochemistry

Despite the widespread use of immunophenotyping in the diagnosis of hematopoietic neoplasms, cytochemical studies are still of diagnostic importance (Scott, 1993). This is particularly true of the acute leukemias, although a large panel of cytochemical tests is probably not necessary in most cases. In rare patients with inconclusive flow cytometry results, cytochemical stains may provide information which can confirm a diagnosis (Mhawech *et al.*, 2001). Myeloperoxidase or Sudan black B cytochemical stains remains the hallmark of a diagnosis of acute myeloid leukemia (AML) in most cases. Some cases, such as minimally differentiated AML and monoblastic leukemias, are myeloperoxidase-negative. The use of non-specific esterase cytochemistry, such as a α-naphthyl butyrate esterase, is still the primary means of identifying monocytic differentiation for classification purposes.

Cytochemistry is of limited value in the diagnosis of acute lymphoblastic leukemia (ALL). Whereas negative results of peroxidase cytochemical studies are expected in ALL, they do not sufficiently exclude a myeloid leukemia and should not be used as the sole evidence of lymphoid lineage. Periodic acid-Schiff staining, frequently showing "block" positivity in lymphoblast cytoplasm, is also not sufficiently specific to confirm a diagnosis.

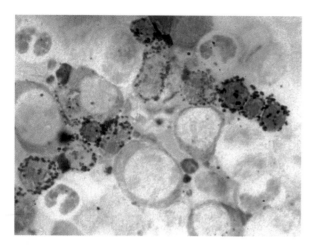

Figure 2.7. An iron stain, illustrating numerous ringed sideroblasts (iron is highlighted as blue granules) in a case of refractory anemia with ringed sideroblasts. Note the perinuclear location of the granules in the erythroid precursors.

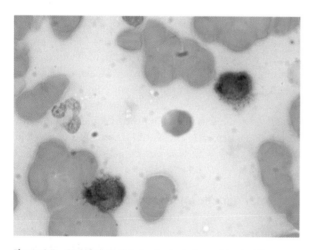

Figure 2.8. Cytochemical stains for tartrate-resistant acid phosphatase (TRAP), demonstrating positivity in circulating hairy cells (hairy cell leukemia).

The Prussian blue stain for iron is a histochemical stain that is commonly employed on bone marrow specimens (Sundberg & Broman, 1955). Although it may be used for clot or biopsy material, it is most reliable and useful for bone marrow aspirate smears, as long as sufficient particles are present on the smear. Iron staining is useful in identifying reticuloendothelial iron stores in the evaluation of a patient for iron deficiency or overload, but it also helps in the evaluation of red blood cell iron incorporation. Iron stores are often graded from 0 to 6+ (Gale *et al.*, 1963), as summarized in Table 2.3, and such grading correlates well with other chemical measures of iron. The identification

of increased iron within erythroid precursors, particularly in the form of ringed sideroblasts, helps in the diagnosis of sideroblastic anemias, myelodysplastic syndromes with ringed sideroblasts, and AML with associated multilineage dysplasia (Fig. 2.7).

The other cytochemical test that is commonly used on bone marrow (and peripheral blood) smears is the detection of tartrate-resistant acid phosphatase (Fig. 2.8) in hairy cell leukemia (HCL) (Yam *et al.*, 1971). At present this cytochemical stain should be used in conjunction with immunophenotypic studies for a complete diagnostic characterization of HCL.

Immunophenotyping

Immunophenotyping studies are essential for the proper diagnosis of lymphoblastic malignant neoplasms, and they help in the classification of mature lymphoid neoplasms and some myeloid neoplasms. In addition, these studies can provide a characteristic immunologic "fingerprint" of an acute leukemia that may be useful in the subsequent evaluation of residual disease.

Some antibodies that are useful in the immunophenotypic evaluation of blastic proliferations by flow cytometry and immunocytochemistry are listed in Table 2.5. The best markers for investigating lymphomas are discussed in Chapter 11.

Both flow cytometry and immunocytochemistry primarily detect surface antigens, although some cytoplasmic and nuclear antigens may also be detected (e.g., CD3 and TdT).

Flow cytometry

Flow cytometry has the advantage of allowing the evaluation of several thousand cells in a rapid manner, and it has the ability to assess the expression of multiple antigens on a single cell. Also, the use of CD45 versus side-scatter gating strategies allows cells with specific characteristics (such as blast cells or lymphoid cells) to be evaluated, and this method greatly increases the ability to detect residual disease in a specimen (Borowitz *et al.*, 1993). Flow cytometry is also the best technique for assessment of clonality in B-cell lymphoid neoplasms (by surface immunoglobulin light chain analysis).

Several consensus reports and reviews regarding the use of flow cytometric immunophenotyping in hematological malignant neoplasms offer guidelines on the use of this methodology on peripheral blood and bone marrow specimens (Rothe & Schmitz, 1996; Borowitz *et al.*, 1997; Braylan *et al.*, 1997; Davis *et al.*, 1997; Jennings & Foon, 1997; Stelzer *et al.*, 1997; Stewart *et al.*, 1997).

Table 2.5. Selected useful flow cytometry and immunocytochemistry markers in acute leukemia.

General
   CD45
Myeloid
   CD11c
   CD13
   CD15
   CD33
   CD65
   CD117
   Cytoplasmic myeloperoxidase
Myelomonocytic
   CD14
   CD36
   CD64
Megakaryocyte
   CD41
   CD61
Immature B lineage
   CD10
   CD19
   CD22
   TdT
Mature B lineage
   CD19
   CD20
   κ and λ light chains
T lineage
   CD2
   CD5
   CD7
   CD4/CD8
   TdT
   Cytoplasmic CD3
Others
   CD34
   CD56
   HLA-DR

Immunohistochemistry

The majority of antibodies that are available for flow cytometry can also be used for immunostaining of paraffin sections of core biopsy or clot material. The main advantages of immunocytochemistry include the direct visualization of the marker on the tumor cell and that it does not require the instrumentation needed for flow cytometry. Disadvantages are a relative lack of standardization, both of the technique and of the reactivity analysis, which frequently limits the reproducibility of the results obtained in different laboratories, and lack of sensitivity with several antigens.

Immunohistochemistry is ideal for the assessment of lesions that are seen in the biopsy but which, due to sampling differences or dry taps, may not be present in the aspirated material submitted for flow cytometry. This includes, in particular, focal marrow involvement by malignant lymphoma and leukemic conditions associated with marrow fibrosis. Immunohistochemistry is also particularly useful for the characterization of tumors that are not routinely assessed by flow cytometry, such as Hodgkin lymphoma, metastatic carcinomas, and small round cell tumors of childhood.

Because of limitations in the detection of some antigens by paraffin section immunohistochemistry and its lesser degree of reproducibility, flow cytometric immunophenotyping is preferred for the evaluation of chronic lymphoproliferative disorders (e.g., chronic lymphocytic leukemia) and acute leukemias. When such material is not available, immunohistochemistry may still provide diagnostic information (Kurec *et al.*, 1990; Arber & Jenkins, 1996; Chuang & Li, 1997; Manaloor *et al.*, 2000). Paraffin section antibodies useful for the evaluation of hematologic malignancies are listed in Table 2.6.

As with all immunophenotyping studies, pertinent positive and negative findings should be obtained with a panel of antibodies because the detection of a single antigen is usually not sufficiently lineage-specific. For example, whereas terminal deoxynucleotidyl transferase (TdT) is usually detectable in lymphoblastic malignant neoplasms (Orazi, 1994), it is also present in a subgroup of myeloid leukemias.

Molecular genetic and cytogenetic analysis

Molecular genetic and cytogenetic studies on bone marrow specimens offer valuable information in certain clinical situations, and the prognostic significance of karyotypic changes in acute leukemia are now well established. In general, routine karyotype analysis is the preferred first-line test in a newly diagnosed case of leukemia or aggressive myelodysplastic syndrome, because a multitude of acquired genetic abnormalities may be detected by this method. When cryptic or masked translocations are suspected, when a precise genetic breakpoint with prognostic implications needs to be confirmed, or when residual disease testing is needed, molecular genetic tests are useful. This testing also helps in identifying gene rearrangements in lymphomas that are not readily identifiable by karyotype analysis and in detecting some lymphoma translocations that may not be consistently found by karyotype analysis. Details about the specific molecular genetic abnormalities

Table 2.6. Selected useful paraffin section antibodies in hematologic malignancies.

Erythroid cells
Hgb
Glycophorin A
Myeloid cells
Myeloperoxidase
Lysozyme
Elastase
CD15
Lactopherrin
CD68
CD43
CD117
Megakaryocytes
Factor VIII antigen (von Willebrand)
CD42b
CD61
Lymphoid cells
B cells
  CD45RB
  CD79a
  CD20
  EMA
  DAB.44
  PAX-5
T cells
  CD3
  CD45RO
  CD4
  CD5
  CD8
NK cells
  CD56
Other
  CD30
  CD34
  TdT
  CD43
Monocytes/macrophages
CD68R
CD68
HAM-56
CD163
Lysozyme
S-100
CD1a

Table 2.7. Some of the common cytogenetic and molecular genetic abnormalities in acute myeloid leukemia and myelodysplasia.

Translocation	Involved genes	Most common Disease type
inv(3)/t(3;3)(q21;q26)	*RPN1/EVI1*	Myelodysplasia
t(3;21)(q26;q22)	*EVI1, or MDS1/AML1*	Myelodysplasia
t(3;5)(q25;q34)	*NPM/MLF1*	Myelodysplasia M2, M6
t(8;21)(q22;q22)	*AML1/ETO*	M2
t(6;9)(p23;q34)	*DEK/CAN*	M1, M2, M4
t(7;11)(p15;p15)	*NUP98/HOXA9*	M2, M4
t(15;17)(q22;q21)	*PML/RARα*	M3
t(11;17)(q23;q21)	*PLZF/RARα*	M3
t(11;17)(q13;q21)	*NuMA/RARα*	M3
t(5;17)(q31;q21)	*NPM/RARα*	M3
inv(16)/t(16;16)(p13;q22)	*CBFβ/MYH11*	M4Eo
t(9;11)(p22;q23)	*AF9/MLL*	M5
Other 11q23 abnormalities	*MLL*	M4, M5
t(1;22)(p13;q31)	*OTT/MAL*	M7

Table 2.8. Some of the common cytogenetic and molecular genetic abnormalities in acute lymphoblastic leukemia.

Type of leukemia	Translocation	Involved genes
Precursor B-Cell ALL (L1, L2)	t(9;22)(q34;q11)	*BCR/ABL*
	t(12;21)(p13;q22)	*TEL/AML1*
	t(1;19)(q23;p13)	*E2A/PBX*
	t(17;19)(q22;p13)	*E2A/HLF*
	t(4;11)(q21;q23)	*AF4/MLL*
	Other 11q23 abnormalities	*MLL*
B-cell ALL (L3)	t(8;14)(q24;q32)	*IGH/MYC*
	t(2;8)(p12;q24)	*IGκ /MYC*
	t(8;22)(q24;q11)	*IGκ /MYC*
T-cell ALL	1q32 abnormalities	*TAL1*
	t(8;14)(q24;q11)	*TCRα/MYC*
	t(11;14)(p15;q11)	*TCRδ/RBTN1*
	t(11;14)(p13;q11)	*TCRδ/RBTN2*
	t(10;14)(p24;q11)	*TCRδ/HOX11*
	del 9(p21)	*p16 and p15*
	t(1;7)(p34;q34)	*TCRβ/LCK*

Tables 2.7 and 2.8. The most common groups of abnormalities are those that disrupt transcription factors, tyrosine kinase translocations, retinoic acid translocations, and 11q23 abnormalities (Sawyers, 1997; Strout & Caligiuri, 1997).

Translocations that involve genes that encode transcription factor proteins are some of the most common in acute leukemia. Of these, the core-binding factor, a transcription

associated with bone marrow diseases are discussed with those diseases in the relevant chapters.

A large number of cytogenetic abnormalities occur with acute leukemias; some of them are summarized in factor involved in normal hematopoiesis, is one of the best described (Downing, 1999). The core-binding factor is formed by an aggregate of different proteins that include the AML1 protein, encoded by the *AML1* gene on chromosome band 21(q22), and the core-binding factor β-subunit protein, which is encoded on chromosome band 16(q22). Disruption of either one of these chromosome regions, as seen in t(8;21), t(3;21), t(12;21), inv(16), and t(16;16), results in the development of acute leukemia or myelodysplasia. These abnormalities may cause loss of the normal transactivation domain on the AML protein or cause disruption of the normal configuration of the core-binding factor. Either mechanism blocks the usual interactions that trigger normal hematopoiesis. The leukemia types of each abnormality vary. The *AML1/ETO* fusion product of t(8;21)(q22;q22) usually results in a *de novo* AML with maturation (M2); *AML1/EVI-1*, *AML1/EAP*, and *AML1/MDS1* fusion products of t(3;21)(q26;q22) are usually seen in myelodysplasia; the *TEL/AML1* fusion of t(12;21)(p13;q22) is associated with pediatric acute lymphoblastic leukemia; and the *CBFβ/MYH11* fusion product of inv(16)(p13q22) or t(16;16)(p13;q22) is usually seen with *de novo* acute myelomonocytic leukemia with abnormal eosinophils (M4Eo). Despite the great variability in the morphologic and immunophenotypic features of these leukemias, they all have a similar molecular genetic mechanism that is at least in part related to the development of the leukemic process.

Translocations resulting in the development of a tyrosine kinase fusion protein are a second group of abnormalities in leukemias. These include the *BCR/ABL* proteins of t(9;22)(q32;q11) in chronic myelogenous leukemia (CML) and some cases of AML, the *TEL/PDGFRβ* protein of t(5;12)(q33;p13) in some cases of chronic myelomonocytic leukemia (CMML), and the *TEL/ABL* fusion protein of t(9;12)(q32;p13) of some acute and chronic leukemias. These tyrosine kinase proteins interact with other proteins to activate the RAS signaling pathway, which may result in abnormal myeloid proliferation.

The t(15;17)(q22;q11.2) is the most common retinoic acid translocation and is present in the majority of acute promyelocytic leukemias. This translocation results in a *PML/RARα* fusion protein. Other less common translocations also occur in acute promyelocytic leukemia and involve the *RARα* gene. Fusion proteins involving *RARα* negatively inhibit the poorly understood normal functions of the *RARα* gene, apparently resulting in the development of acute leukemia. This mechanism of leukemia transformation is unique to the acute promyelocytic leukemias. All-*trans*-retinoic acid overrides the negative inhibitory effect of the leukemic fusion protein, making it a unique therapeutic agent for the disease.

Translocations involving chromosome band 11q23 are common, and at least 30 different translocation partners may occur with the chromosome region in acute leukemia. Most translocations involve the *MLL* gene that is also known as *ALL1* and *HRX* (DiMartino & Cleary, 1999). The *MLL* gene is believed to function as a homeostatic transcription regulator, but how translocations involving this gene cause leukemia are not well understood. The type of leukemia differs with the different *MLL* translocations. The t(4;11)(q21;q23) results in an *AF4/MLL* fusion protein. This translocation is usually associated with precursor B-cell ALL, often with aberrant CD15 and CD65 expression, and is extremely common in infants. The t(9;11)(p22;q23) results in an *AF9/MLL* fusion protein and is more commonly associated with AMLs in adults with monocytic features. Translocations involving the *MLL* and *AML1* genes also occur in therapy-related AMLs and are common after chemotherapy with topoisomerase II inhibitors. The *MLL* leukemias also usually demonstrate monocytic features, but may also present as therapy-related acute lymphoblastic leukemias.

The lymphoid malignant neoplasms also demonstrate evidence of immunoglobulin or T-cell receptor gene rearrangements that may be useful markers of clonality. Such tests are usually not necessary to make a diagnosis of malignancy in cases of acute leukemia, and because lineage infidelity is common in ALLs these tests may not be useful in defining cell lineage. A unique gene rearrangement in an ALL may be sequenced, however, and patient-specific polymerase chain reaction (PCR) primers and probes, which have been shown to be useful for the monitoring of residual disease, may be developed. These methods are not available in most medical centers for routine use. The mature lymphoid malignant neoplasms also demonstrate gene rearrangements, and many are associated with unique cytogenetic translocations. These are discussed in more detail with each disease and in Chapter 11.

Cytogenetic studies are essential to identify the abnormality associated with a given leukemia, although t(12;21) and some *MLL* translocations may be missed by routine karyotype analysis. PCR methods are useful for confirming a precise translocation site and are potentially useful in following up patients for residual disease. Some translocations, including t(8;21) and possibly inv(16), may persist in low numbers after treatment. Detection of these abnormalities by routine PCR methods does not necessarily predict relapse. For this reason, quantitative PCR methods may be of more value in the future for the detection of residual disease after therapy (Yin & Tobal, 1999).

Table 2.9. Elements to include in a bone marrow report.

Clinical indication for bone marrow study
Peripheral blood examination
  Complete blood count data including reticulocyte count
  Red blood cell changes
    Red blood cell number and size
    Hypochromasia, if present
    Description of anisocytosis and poikilocytosis and description of granules or inclusions, if present
    Presence of increased polychromasia, if present
  White blood cell changes
    White blood cell number
    Description of cell types with relative hyperplasias, cytopenias, or left shift
    Description of dysplastic or toxic changes
    Presence or absence of blast cells, atypical or neoplastic lymphoid cells, or other abnormal cell populations
  Platelet changes
    Platelet number
    Platelet morphology, including granulation and size
Bone marrow aspirate smear or imprint
  Adequacy
  Relative cellularity (hypo, moderate, hypercellular)
  Myeloid-to-erythroid ratio
  Red blood cell precursors
    Relative percentage
    Normal maturation versus left shift
    Dysplastic changes
  Granulocyte precursors
    Relative percentage
    Normal maturation versus left shift
    Dysplastic changes
    Percentage of blasts and description of blasts if evaluated
  Megakaryocytes
    Relative number
    Description of morphology, including size and nuclear features
  Description of other cell types, including evaluations of lymphocytes, plasma cells, monocytes, mast cells,
    eosinophils, and basophils
  Differential cell count (typically 300 or 500 cell), if indicated
Bone marrow trephine or clot biopsy
  Adequacy
  Marrow cellularity, including percentage and comparison to normal cellularity for age
  Proportions of myeloid to erythroid cells
  Relative number of megakaryocytes
  Features of bone trabeculae
  Degree of fibrosis, if present
  Abnormal cellular infiltrates, including granulomas, lymphoid cell infiltrates, plasma cells, and metastatic tumor
    Percentage of marrow involvement
    Location and pattern (particularly neoplastic lymphoid infiltrates)
    Cell type (lymphoma cell type or differentiation of plasma cell infiltrate)
Cytochemistry results, if indicated
  Iron stain results for reticuloendothelial stores and red blood cell incorporation, including presence and percentage
    of ringed sideroblasts
  Cytochemical studies for acute leukemia or hairy cell leukemia, including stains performed and results

(cont.)

Table 2.9. (*cont.*)

Immunophenotyping results, if indicated

    Method used (e.g., flow cytometry, immunocytochemistry, immunohistochemistry)

    Antibodies and antigens studied

    Cell population studies (e.g., blast cells, lymphoid cells, plasma cells)

    Specimen type studies (peripheral blood, bone marrow aspirate, bone marrow biopsy)

    Results for each antibody and antigen and interpretation of total findings

Molecular genetic and cytogenetic studies, if indicated

    Method used (e.g., karyotype analysis, polymerase chain reaction, Southern blot, fluorescence *in situ* hybridization)

    Test performed (e.g., *BCR/ABL*, RT-PCR, or FISH, immunoglobulin heavy chain gene rearrangement PCR)

    Interpretation of results

Diagnosis

    Tissue examined

    Diagnostic interpretation, incorporating all results

    Classification system used clearly indicated in the diagnosis (if in question)

The bone marrow report

Table 2.9 lists the suggested elements to include in the bone marrow report. Many elements of the report, as well as which tests are performed, are determined by the initial morphologic findings and clinical situation; the clinical indication for the bone marrow examination should therefore be included. Available complete blood cell count data should also be included as well as review of the peripheral blood smear. Adequacy or inadequacy of the sample also should be commented upon.

The bone marrow aspirate and biopsy examinations describe the three main cell lineages of the marrow and, as appropriate, other cellular elements. In the case of infiltrative lesions in the marrow, the cell type and percentage of involvement are included. Results of all ancillary studies are ideally included in the final report and correlated with the final diagnosis. This may require amending the report when ancillary study results that are not available at the time of the initial report, such as molecular genetic or cytogenetic results, become available. This multi-step approach allows for a final "comprehensive" diagnostic interpretation that is based on all available data and addresses all findings, including seemingly contradictory data that may be easily explained when all of the information is considered together.

REFERENCES

Arber, D. A. & Jenkins, K. A. (1996). Paraffin section immunophenotyping of acute leukemias in bone marrow specimens. *American Journal of Clinical Pathology*, **106**, 462–8.

Bain, B. J. (1996). The normal bone marrow. In *Bone Marrow Pathology*, 2nd edn., ed. B. J. Bain, D. M. Clark, & I. A. Lampert. Oxford: Blackwell, pp. 1–50.

Borowitz, M. J., Guenther, K. L., Shults, K. E., & Stelzer, G. T. (1993). Immunophenotyping of acute leukemia by flow cytometric analysis: use of CD45 and right-angle light scatter to gate on leukemic blasts in three-color analysis. *American Journal of Clinical Pathology*, **100**, 534–40.

Borowitz, M. J., Bray, R., Gascoyne, R., *et al.* (1997). US–Canadian consensus recommendations on the immunophenotypic analysis of hematologic neoplasia by flow cytometry: data analysis and interpretation. *Cytometry*, **30**, 236–44.

Braylan, R. C., Atwaiter, S. K., Diamond, L., *et al.* (1997). US–Canadian consensus recommendations on the immunophenotypic analysis of hematologic neoplasia by flow cytometry: data reporting. *Cytometry*, **30**, 245–8.

Brown, D. C. & Gatter, K. C. (1993). The bone marrow trephine biopsy: a review of normal histology. *Histopathology*, **22**, 411–22.

Cattoretti, G., Schiro, R., Orazi, A., Soligo, D., & Colombo, M. P. (1993). Bone marrow stroma in humans: anti-nerve growth factors receptor antibodies selectively stain reticular cells in vivo and in vitro. *Blood*, **81**, 1726–38.

Chuang, S. S. & Li, C. Y. (1997). Useful panel of antibodies for the classification of acute leukemia by immunohistochemical methods in bone marrow trephine biopsy specimens. *American Journal of Clinical Pathology*, **107**, 410–18.

Davis, B. H., Foucar, K., Szczarkowski, W., *et al.* (1997). US–Canadian consensus recommendations on the immunophenotypic analysis of hematologic neoplasia by flow cytometry: medical indications. *Cytometry*, **30**, 249–63.

DiMartino, J. F. & Cleary, M. L. (1999). MLL rearrangements in hematological malignancies: lessons from clinical and biological studies. *British Journal of Haematology*, **106**, 614–24.

Downing, J. R. (1999). The AML1-ETO chimaeric transcription factor in acute myeloid leukaemia: biology and clinical significance. *British Journal of Haematology*, **106**, 296–308.

Fong, T. P., Okafor, L. A., Schmitz, T. H., Thomas, W., & Westerman, M. P. (1979). An evaluation of cellularity in various types of bone marrow specimens. *American Journal of Clinical Pathology*, **72**, 812–16.

Foucar, K. (2001). *Bone Marrow Pathology*, 2nd edn. Chicago, IL: ASCP Press.

Friebert, S. E., Shepardson, L. B., Shurin, S. B., Rosenthal, G. E., & Rosenthal, N. S. (1998). Pediatric bone marrow cellularity: are we expecting too much? *Journal of Pediatric Hematology/Oncology*, **20**, 439–43.

Frisch, B. & Bartl, R. (1999). *Biopsy Interpretation of Bone and Bone Marrow: Histology and Immunohistology in Paraffin and Plastic*. London: Arnold.

Gale, E., Torrance, J., & Bothwell, T. (1963). The quantitative estimation of total iron stores in human bone marrow. *Journal of Clinical Investigation*, **42**, 1076–82.

Gruppo, R. A., Lampkin, B. C., & Granger, S. (1997). Bone marrow cellularity determination: comparison of the biopsy, aspirate, and buffy coat. *Blood*, **49**, 29–31.

Gulati, G. L., Ashton, J. K., & Hyun, B. H. (1988). Structure and function of the bone marrow and hematopoiesis. *Hematology/Oncology Clinics of North America*, **2**, 495–511.

Hartsock, R. J., Smith, E. B., & Petty, C. S. (1965). Normal variations with aging of the amount of hematopoietic tissue in bone marrow from the anterior iliac crest: a study made from 177 cases of sudden death necropsy. *American Journal of Clinical Pathology*, **43**, 326–31.

Jennings, C. D. & Foon, K. A. (1997). Recent advances in flow cytometry: application to the diagnosis of hematologic malignancy. *Blood*, **90**, 2863–92.

Kurec, A. S., Cruz, V. E., Barrett, D., Mason, D. Y., & Davey, F. R. (1990). Immunophenotyping of acute leukemias using paraffin-embedded tissue sections. *American Journal of Clinical Pathology*, **93**, 502–9.

Longacre, T. A., Foucar, K., Crago, S., *et al.* (1989). Hematogones: a multiparameter analysis of bone marrow precursor cells. *Blood*, **73**, 544–52.

Manaloor, E. J., Neiman, R. S., Heilman, D. K., *et al.* (2000). IHC of routinely processed bone marrow biopsies can be used to subtype AML: comparison with flow cytometry. *American Journal of Clinical Pathology*, **113**, 814–22.

Manoharan, A., Horsley, R., & Pitney, W. R. (1979). The reticulin content of bone marrow in acute leukemia in adults. *British Journal of Haematology*, **43**, 185–90.

Mhawech, P., Buffone, G. J., Khan, S. P., & Gresik, M. V. (2001). Cytochemical staining and flow cytometry methods applied to the diagnosis of acute leukemia in the pediatric population: an assessment of relative usefulness. *Journal of Pediatric Hematology/Oncology*, **23**, 89–92.

Naeim, F. (1998). *Pathology of Bone Marrow*. Baltimore, MD: Williams & Wilkins.

Orazi, A., Cotton, J., Cattoretti, G., *et al.* (1994). Terminal deoxnucleotidyl transferase staining in acute leukemia and normal bone marrow in routinely processed paraffin sections. *American Journal of Clinical Pathology*, **102**, 640–5.

Rothe, G. & Schmitz, G. (1996). Consensus protocol for the flow cytometric immunotyping of hematopoietic malignancies. *Leukemia*, **10**, 877–95.

Sawyers, C. L. (1997). Molecular genetics of acute leukemia. *Lancet*, **349**, 196–200.

Scott, C. S., Den Ottolander, G. J., Swirsky, D., *et al.* (1993). Recommended procedures for the classification of acute leukaemia. *Leukemia and Lymphoma*, **11**, 37–49.

Stelzer, G. T., Marti, G., Hurley, A., McCoy, P. Jr., Lovett, E. J., & Schwartz, A. (1997). US–Canadian consensus recommendations on the immunophenotypic analysis of hematologic neoplasia by flow cytometry: standardization and validation of laboratory procedures. *Cytometry*, **30**, 214–30.

Stewart, C. C., Behm, F. G., Carey, J. L., *et al.* (1997). US–Canadian consensus recommendations on the immunophenotypic analysis of hematologic neoplasia by flow cytometry: selection of antibody combinations. *Cytometry*, **30**, 231–5.

Strauchen, J. A. (1996). *Diagnostic Histopathology of the Bone Marrow*. New York, NY: Oxford University Press.

Strout, M. P. & Caligiuri, M. A. (1997). Developments in cytogenetics and oncogenes in acute leukemia. *Current Opinion in Oncology*, **9**, 8–17.

Sundberg, R. D. & Broman, H. (1955). The application of the Prussian blue stain to previously stained films of blood and bone marrow. *Blood*, **10**, 160–6.

Teitelbaum, S. L. & Bullough, P. G. (1979). The pathophysiology of bone and joint disease. *American Journal of Pathology*, **96**, 282–354.

Yam, L. T., Li, C. Y., & Lam, K. W. (1971). Tartrate-resistant acid phosphatase isoenzyme in the reticulum cells of leukemic reticuloendotheliosis. *New England Journal of Medicine*, **284**, 357–60.

Yin, J. A. & Tobal, K. (1999). Detection of minimal residual disease in acute myeloid leukaemia: methodologies, clinical and biological significance. *British Journal of Haematology*, **106**, 578–90.

3

Granulomatous and histiocytic disorders

Granulomas in bone marrow

Although aggregates of histiocytes may be present on aspirate smears, granulomas are best identified with bone marrow trephine and clot biopsy materials (Bodem *et al.*, 1983; Bhargava & Farhi, 1988; Vilalta-Castel *et al.*, 1988; Foucar, 2001; Chang *et al.*, 2003). Granulomas in the bone marrow should be approached in a similar fashion to those in other sites.

There are generally two types of granulomas encountered in the marrow. The lipogranuloma is a collection of histiocytes surrounding adipose tissue and is usually not associated with disease (Rywlin & Ortega, 1972) (Fig. 3.1). Epithelioid granulomas without associated adipose tissue may have admixed lymphocytes, plasma cells, neutrophils, or eosinophils and may have associated necrosis (Fig. 3.2). Mycobacteria and fungal organisms should be excluded by special stains in all cases with epithelioid granulomas, and fresh bone marrow aspirate material should be submitted for culture in all patients being evaluated for infectious diseases.

The most common causes of infectious granulomas are summarized in Table 3.1. Patients with immunodeficiency syndromes may have a disseminated atypical mycobacterial infection caused by *Mycobacterium avium–intracellulare* (MAI) even when well-formed granulomas are not present. In such cases, special stains for organisms are indicated when any increase in histiocytes is noted. MAI may also be associated with the presence of "pseudo-Gaucher" macrophages in which the intracellular organisms mimic the characteristic cytoplasmic striations of Gaucher cells. MAI shows a characteristic periodic acid-Schiff (PAS) positivity, while in tuberculosis the organisms are usually PAS-negative (Fig. 3.3). In addition, MAI is also stained by acid-fast bacilli (AFB) as well as Grocott methanamine silver (GMS) techniques.

Marrow involved by leprosy can show a diffuse proliferation of foamy macrophages while well-formed granulomas are lacking (Strauchen, 1996). Although fungi and mycobacteria are the most common infectious causes of bone marrow granulomas, various bacterial and viral infections may also cause them (Table 3.1). Occasional infectious granulomas, particularly those associated with Q fever, brucellosis, and ehrlichiosis contain a central clear space surrounded by fibrin that may be mistaken for an incidental lipogranuloma (Srigley *et al.*, 1985). Similar "fibrin ring granulomas" have also been described with cytomegalovirus infection (Young & Goulian, 1993).

Non-infectious causes of granulomas (Table 3.2), which include sarcoidosis, drug reactions, collagen–vascular disease, and neoplasm-associated, cannot be reliably distinguished from infectious granulomas, and appropriate histochemical stains for organisms are indicated in these patients (Fig. 3.4). Bone marrow granulomas are common in patients with Hodgkin lymphoma and non-Hodgkin lymphomas and may be present both in the presence and in the absence of bone marrow involvement by the neoplasm (Yu & Rywlin, 1982). Although non-infectious granulomas are more common, most of these patients are also at risk for the development of infection-associated granulomas. In Hodgkin lymphoma, multiple step sections through the biopsy specimen should be examined before a diagnosis of granulomas without involvement by Hodgkin lymphoma is made, because only rare Hodgkin cells may be present in the specimen.

The findings of epithelioid granulomas have been widely reported in Hodgkin lymphoma and peripheral T-cell lymphoma (e.g., Lennert lymphoma). Similar granulomas can occur in B-cell lymphomas and may also cause diagnostic confusion. In those cases, immunohistology may be very helpful in highlighting subtle involvement of the marrow with lymphoma.

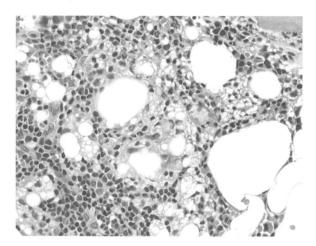

Figure 3.1. Lipogranuloma. Note the multilobulated appearance of the adipocytes. Lymphocytes are seen associated with the lipogranuloma.

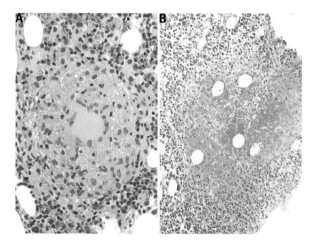

Figure 3.2. (A) An epithelioid granuloma. Note the large pink-staining macrophages and, in this case, a Langerhans-type giant cell. Note also the rim of lymphocytes around the granuloma. (B) Granuloma with central necrosis in a case of miliary tuberculosis.

Hemophagocytic syndromes

Hemophagocytic syndrome may be a primary or secondary disorder. Primary hemophagocytic lymphohistiocytosis is a rare, fatal childhood disorder that may be familial or sporadic (Arico *et al.*, 1996). It is usually elicited by a viral infection, and in some cases is due to germline mutations of perforin, *SH2D1A* or other genes (Stepp *et al.*, 1999; Arico *et al.*, 2001). Bone marrow involvement may be evident in only 40% of cases that have extensive disease elsewhere (Ost *et al.*, 1998). Secondary hemophagocytosis may be

Table 3.1. Causes of infectious granulomas in the bone marrow.

Bacterial/rickettsial	
	Brucellosis
	Tularemia
	Rocky Mountain spotted fever
	Q fever
	Mycoplasma pneumoniae
Mycobacterial	
	Mycobacterium tuberculosis
	M. avium-intracellulare (MAI)
	Bacillus Calmette–Guerin (BCG)
	M. leprae
	Atypical mycobacteria
Fungal	
	Histoplasma
	Cryptococcus
	Coccidioidomycosis
	Saccharomyces
	Aspergillus spp.
Protozoal/parasitic	
	Toxoplasmosis
	Leishmania
Viral	
	Epstein–Barr virus (EBV)
	Cytomegalovirus (CMV)
	Viral hepatitis (Hepatitis C, others)

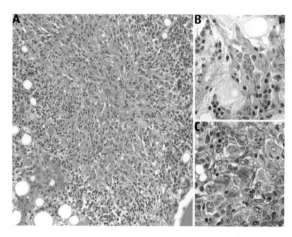

Figure 3.3. Granuloma associated with *Mycobacterium avium–intracellulare* (MAI). Note (A) the relatively ill-formed nature of the granuloma, (B) numerous AFB-positive organisms and (C) organisms positive for PAS, a feature not seen in *M. tuberculosis*.

infectious or neoplasia-related (McKenna *et al.*, 1981; Risdall *et al.*, 1984; Takeshita *et al.*, 1993).

All types frequently involve multiple organs, including the bone marrow, and have similar morphologic features

Table 3.2. Diseases associated with bone marrow granulomas that may not be infection-related.

Cause	Comments
Neoplasms	
Hodgkin lymphoma	Often see granulomas in absence of lymphomatous infiltrate
Non-Hodgkin lymphoma	May see granulomas admixed with overt lymphoma
Acute and chronic leukemias	Admixed with leukemic infiltrates
Carcinomas	
Myelodysplasias	Granulomas rarely noted in these patients
Other disorders/conditions	
Immune disorders	Rheumatoid arthritis, systemic lupus erythematosus, other autoimmune processes
Sarcoidosis	Very rare to have bone marrow granulomas in absence of pulmonary disease
BCG therapy	Elicits granulomatous response in bone marrow
Drug reactions	Uncommon finding: described in patients receiving a variety of treatments including procainamide, sulfonamides, amiodarone
Pneumoconiosis/silicosis	May see associated pigment/silica
HIV/AIDS	Infectious granulomas are also common in these groups

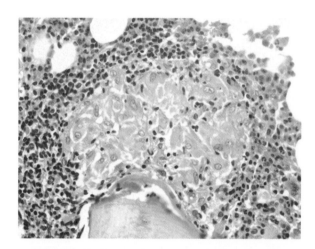

Figure 3.4. A sarcoid-type granuloma. Sarcoidal granulomas seen in bone marrow and other sites have a "hard" appearance with sharply defined borders. Note also the surrounding rim of small lymphocytes.

(Fig. 3.5). Hemophagocytosis consists, most prominently, of erythrophagocytosis that may be better visualized on aspirate smears or imprint slides. The histiocytes have characteristically bland nuclear features without mitosis or atypia. Other marrow elements, particularly granulocytes and erythroid precursors, may be relatively decreased in number. Reactive lymphoid cells, immunoblasts in particular, may be increased in the marrow in association with hemophagocytosis. The presence of immunoblasts does not necessarily indicate the presence of an associated

lymphoma. The possibility of a viral etiology, Epstein–Barr virus (EBV) in particular, should be ruled out in these cases by immunostaining the section with EBV-LMP and/or by *in situ* analysis (e.g., EBER1 RNA). Cytologic atypia of the lymphoid cells should be easily identified in lymphoma-associated hemophagocytosis. In reactive cases, the majority of the lymphoid cells often consist of CD8-positive small T lymphocytes. Gene rearrangement studies may be helpful in making a primary diagnosis of lymphoma on a bone marrow specimen with extensive hemophagocytosis.

Hemophagocytosis may be associated with T-cell malignant neoplasms, and many of these cases in the past were interpreted as malignant histiocytosis. The neoplastic T cells are usually distinct from the reactive-appearing histiocytes that are engulfing other hematopoietic cells; this may include phagocytosis of neoplastic cells. In some cases, the bone marrow may demonstrate evidence of hemophagocytosis without definite marrow involvement by the T-cell neoplasm that is prominent in other sites.

Storage diseases

Various storage diseases may involve the bone marrow, and should be diagnosed and classified by identification of the enzymatic defect characteristic of each disease (Scriver *et al.*, 1995). Gaucher and Niemann–Pick diseases are the most common storage diseases encountered in the bone marrow, and both may cause the accumulation of patchy or diffuse aggregates of large histiocytes with abundant cytoplasm and small nuclei (Volk *et al.*, 1972) (Fig. 3.6). On smears, Gaucher cells have slightly basophilic cytoplasm

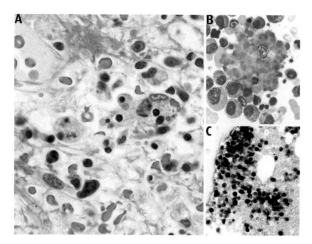

Figure 3.5. Infection-associated hemophagocytic syndrome. (A) Section of core biopsy shows a hypocellular bone marrow containing numerous macrophages with ingested cellular elements. (B) A bone marrow aspirate smear with a macrophage which has ingested numerous erythrocytes. (C) Epstein–Barr virus *in situ* hybridization for EBER showing nuclear positivity for EBV mRNA in marrow lymphocytes.

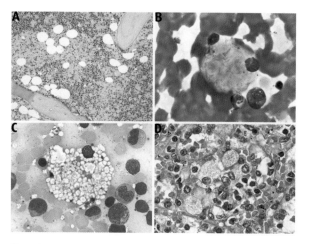

Figure 3.6. (A) Bone marrow involvement by Gaucher disease. Note the foamy macrophages in the interstitial spaces forming large aggregates. (B) High magnification of a Gaucher cell seen in an aspirate smear. Note the classic "folded tissue paper" appearance of the striated cytoplasm. Bone marrow involvement in Niemann–Pick disease: (C) Aspirate smear showing a large multi-vacuolated macrophage. (D) Characteristic multi-vacuolated macrophages, in this case seen in an H&E-stained section of spleen.

that is often compared with crumpled tissue paper, in contrast to the finely vacuolated cytoplasm of the characteristic cells of Niemann–Pick disease (Fig. 3.6).

Characteristic Gaucher cells range in size from 20 to 100 μm in diameter and have fibrillar cytoplasm that appears brownish in H&E-stained preparations. Multinucleated cells may occur. The cytoplasm is intensely PAS-positive, and the PAS positivity is resistant to diastase digestion. The glucocerebroside in Gaucher cells is autofluorescent. Because Gaucher cells are macrophages and ingest red blood cells, they may frequently stain positively for iron. Lipid stains are only weakly positive. Ultrastructural studies reveal numerous lysosomes containing characteristic lipid bilayers.

Niemann–Pick cells are large, ranging from 20 to 100 μm in diameter, and appear foamy or bubbly owing to numerous small vacuoles. They are clearer than Gaucher cells and usually stain only faintly with the PAS stain but contain neutral fat as demonstrated by Sudan black B and oil red O stains. The lipid deposits are birefringent and, under ultraviolet light, display yellow-green fluorescence. Electron microscopy reveals lamellated structures resembling myelin figures within lysosomes. Smaller histiocytes with more basophilic cytoplasm and vacuoles stain blue-green with Romanovsky and are often termed sea-blue histiocytes; they are seen characteristically in cases of ceroid histiocytosis but can also be seen in Niemann–Pick disease. Ceroid-containing histiocytes measure up to

20 μm and contain cytoplasmic granules that measure 3–4 μm. The histiocytes show a variable degree of granulation. Foamy histiocytes with smaller, darker granules may also occur. Ceroid is composed of phospholipids and glycosphingolipids, and is similar to lipofuscin in its physical and chemical properties. Histiocytes containing ceroid appear faintly yellow-brown in H&E-stained sections. Ceroid is PAS-positive and resistant to diastase digestion, and stains positively with lipid stains. It shows a strong affinity for basic dyes such as fuchsin and methylene blue. Ceroid is acid-fast and becomes autofluorescent with aging of the pigment. Ultrastructural studies reveal inclusions of lamellated membranous material with 4.5–5 nm periodicity. None of these cell types is specific for a given disease, and sea-blue histiocytes may also be seen in association with lipid disorders, infectious diseases, red blood cell disorders, and myeloproliferative disorders. Therefore, the accumulation of histiocytes of these types may suggest a storage disease, but the actual diagnosis should be based on biochemical or molecular genetic testing specific for these diseases.

Pseudo-Gaucher cells are often seen in marrows of patients with chronic myelogenous leukemia. Studies have shown (Florena *et al.*, 1996) that Gaucher cells and pseudo-Gaucher cells express a very similar immunophenotype

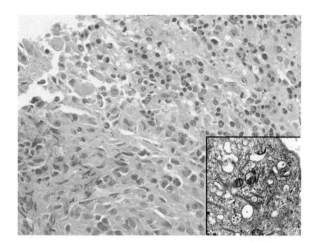

Figure 3.7. Langerhans cell histiocytosis (formerly called histiocytosis X). Note the numerous elongated macrophages with prominent associated eosinophilia. The macrophages often have distinct nuclear grooves. (*Inset*) Electron micrograph showing classic Birbeck granules, an ultrastructural feature diagnostic for Langerhans cell histiocytosis.

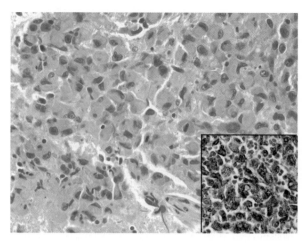

Figure 3.8. Histiocytic sarcoma in bone marrow. The H&E section shows numerous large mature-appearing macrophages present in sheets in the bone marrow. (*Inset*) CD68 stain on a similar case, showing diffuse positivity in the histiocytes/macrophages.

and display an intense reaction for the monocytic antibodies tested, thus confirming their similarities.

Non-leukemic histiocytic disorders

Histiocytic disorders, other than acute and chronic leukemias, are rare in the bone marrow. Langerhans cell histiocytosis, sinus histiocytosis with massive lymphadenopathy, and histiocytic sarcoma (true histiocytic lymphoma) generally present in other organs and only rarely and focally involve the marrow. Langerhans cell histiocytosis, also known as histiocytosis X, is a disease with various clinical presentations that shows an increase in histiocytic cells with grooved nuclei as well as admixed eosinophils. The cells characteristically express CD1a by immunohistochemistry and show Birbeck granules by electron microscopy (Fig. 3.7).

Bone marrow involvement by histiocytic sarcoma, also known as malignant histiocytosis or true histiocytic lymphoma, is controversial. Most cases seem to represent acute monoblastic leukemia without obvious peripheral blood involvement, or cases of monoblastic myeloid sarcoma with minimal or no evidence of bone marrow involvement (Elghetany, 1997; Favara *et al.*, 1997) (Fig. 3.8). Cases of hemophagocytic syndrome (with or without associated malignant disease), anaplastic large cell lymphoma, and other malignant lymphomas with bone marrow involvement have previously been interpreted as malignant histi-

ocytosis (Wilson *et al.*, 1990). Because of the historic heterogeneity of diseases covered by this term, as well as the current lack of specific features that distinguish malignant histiocytosis of the bone marrow from acute monoblastic leukemia, we recommend restricting the use of this term to secondary bone marrow involvement in patients with histiocytic sarcoma (Bucsky & Egeler, 1998).

Rare cases of disseminated histiocytic sarcoma involving, among other organs, the bone marrow have been reported in patients with mediastinal germ cell tumors (Orazi *et al.*, 1993). Immunophenotypically, histiocytic sarcoma cases express histiocyte-associated markers (CD68, CD163, lysozyme, alpha-1-antitrypsin), CD45, or CD45RO, and are negative for CD1a, epithelial, and B- and T-cell lineage-specific markers. Reactivity for S-100 is observed in a variable proportion of cells in these cases (Copie-Bergman *et al.*, 1998). Gene rearrangement analyses for T- and B-cell genes are negative.

REFERENCES

Arico, M., Janka, G., Fischer, A., *et al* (1996). Hemophagocytic lymphohistiocytosis: report of 122 children from the International Registry. *Leukemia*, **10**, 197–203.

Arico, M., Imashuku, S., Clementi, R., *et al*. (2001). Hemophagocytic lymphohistiocytosis due to germline mutations in *SH2D1A*, the X-linked lymphoproliferative disease gene. *Blood*, **97**, 1131–3.

Bhargava, V. & Farhi, D.C. (1988). Bone marrow granulomas: clinicopathologic findings in 72 cases and review of the literature. *Hematologic Pathology*, **21**, 44–50.

Bodem, C. R., Hamory, B. H., Taylor, H. M., & Kleopfer L. (1983). Granulomatous bone marrow disease: a review of the literature and clinicopathologic analysis of 58 cases. *Medicine (Baltimore)*, **62**, 372–83.

Bucsky, P. & Egeler, R. M. (1998). Malignant histiocytic disorders in children: clinical and therapeutic approaches with a nosologic discussion. *Hematology/Oncology Clinics of North America*, **12**, 465–71.

Chang, K. L., Gaal, K. K., Huang, Q., & Weiss, L. M. (2003). Histiocytic lesions involving the bone marrow. *Seminars in Diagnostic Pathology*, **20**, 226–36.

Copie-Bergman, C., Wotherspoon, A. C., Norton, A. J., Diss, T. C., & Isaacson, P. G. (1998). True histiocytic lymphoma: a morphologic, immunohistochemical, and molecular genetic study of 13 cases. *American Journal of Surgical Pathology*, **22**, 1386–92.

Elghetany, M. T. (1997). True histiocytic lymphoma: is it an entity? *Leukemia*, **11**, 762–4.

Favara, B. E., Feller, A. C., Pauli, M., *et al.* (1997). Contemporary classification of histiocytic disorders. *Medical and Pediatric Oncology*, **29**, 157–66.

Florena, A. M., Franco, V., & Campesi G. (1996). Immunophenotypical comparison of Gaucher's and pseudo-Gaucher cells. *Pathology International*, **46**, 155–60.

Foucar, K. (2001). Miscellaneous disorders of the bone marrow, including stromal and bone abnormalities. In *Bone Marrow Pathology*, 2nd edn, Chicago IL: ASCP Press, pp. 564–9.

McKenna, R. W., Risdall, R. J., & Brunning, R. D. (1981). Virus associated hemophagocytic syndrome. *Human Pathology*, **12**, 395–8.

Orazi, A., Neiman, R. S., Ulbright, T. M., Heerema, N. A., John, K., & Nichols, C. R. (1993). Hematopoietic precursor cells within the yolk sac tumor component are the source of secondary hematopoietic malignancies in patients with mediastinal germ cell tumors. *Cancer*, **71**, 3873–81.

Ost, A., Nilsson-Ardnor, S., & Henter, J. I. (1998). Autopsy findings in 27 children with haemophagocytic lymphohistiocytosis. *Histopathology*, **32**, 310–16.

Risdall, R. J., Brunning, R. D., Hernandez, J. I., & Gordon, D. H. (1984). Bacterial-associated hemophagocytic syndrome. *Cancer*, **54**, 2968–72.

Rywlin A. M. & Ortega R. (1972). Lipid granulomas of the bone marrow. *American Journal of Clinical Pathology*, **57**, 457–62.

Scriver, C. R., Beaudet, A. L., Sly, W. S., & Valle, D. (1995). *The Metabolic and Molecular Bases of Inherited Disease*, 7th edn. New York, NY: McGraw-Hill.

Srigley, J. R., Vellend, H., Palmer, N., *et al.* (1985). Q-fever: the liver and bone marrow pathology. *American Journal of Surgical Pathology*, **9**, 752–8.

Stepp, S. E., Dufourcq-Lagelouse, R., Le Deist, F., *et al.* (1999). Perforin gene defects in familial hemophagocytic lymphohistiocytosis. *Science*, **286**, 1957–9.

Strauchen, J. A. (1996). *Diagnostic Histopathology of the Bone Marrow*. New York, NY: Oxford University Press.

Takeshita, M., Kikuchi, M., Ohshima, K., *et al.* (1993). Bone marrow findings in malignant histiocytosis and/or malignant lymphoma with concurrent hemophagocytic syndrome. *Leukemia and Lymphoma*, **12**, 79–89.

Vilalta-Castel, E., Valdes-Sanchez, M. D., Teno-Esteban, C., *et al.* (1988). Significance of granulomas in bone marrow: a study of 40 cases. *European Journal of Haematology*, **41**, 12–16.

Volk, B. W., Adachi, M., & Schneck, L. (1972). The pathology of sphingolipidoses. *Seminars in Hematology*, **9**, 317–48.

Wilson, M. S., Weiss, L. M., Gatter, K. C., Mason, D. Y., Dorfman, R. F., & Warnke, R. A. (1990). Malignant histiocytosis: a reassessment of cases previously reported in 1975 based on paraffin section immunophenotyping studies. *Cancer*, **66**, 530–6.

Young, J. R. & Goulian, M. (1993). Bone marrow fibrin ring granulomas and cytomegalovirus infection. *American Journal of Clinical Pathology*, **99**, 65–8.

Yu, H. C. & Rywlin, A. M. (1982). Granulomatous lesions of the bone marrow in non-Hodgkin's lymphoma. *Human Pathology*, **13**, 905–10.

4

The aplasias

Introduction

A decrease in bone marrow cellularity for a patient's age may be related to a variety of causes. Artifactual hypocellularity due to sampling of only subcortical marrow should not be misinterpreted, and an accurate estimate of marrow cellularity cannot be made on small biopsy specimens that contain only the subcortical marrow space. True hypocellularity may be due to a decrease in all marrow cell lines or decreases in only selected cell lines.

Aplastic anemia

Aplastic anemia (AA) may be acquired or constitutional (congenital), and represents a decrease in granulocytic, erythroid, and megakaryocytic cells (Guinan, 1997; Young, 1999). The principal conditions associated with the development of acquired and inherited aplastic anemia are summarized in Table 4.1.

Diagnostic criteria for severe aplastic anemia are (1) a bone marrow of less than 25% of normal age-related cellularity values, and (2) two of the following three peripheral blood findings: a neutrophil count of less than 0.5×10^9/L, a platelet count of less than 20×10^9/L, anemia with a corrected reticulocyte count of less than 1%. A grading system for AA patients is summarized in Table 4.2.

The peripheral blood demonstrates pancytopenia without obvious abnormalities of the circulating cells (Camitta et al., 1979). Aspirate smears usually show small particles containing histiocytes, mast cells, lymphocytes, and plasma cells with no or rare normal hematopoietic cells. The biopsy specimens in these patients are variably hypocellular (Fig. 4.1). Some have only rare hematopoietic cells, representing less than 5% of the marrow cellularity; others have large areas of markedly hypocellular marrow

admixed with more normocellular areas. Interstitial small lymphocytes, as well as well-formed lymphoid aggregates, are common. Marrow plasmacytosis may be conspicuous, particularly in cases of AA associated with autoimmune/collagen disorders (e.g., lupus). Fibrosis is absent in most cases of aplastic anemia.

Aplastic marrow may be seen after toxic exposures (e.g., benzene, insecticides, and solvents) or viral infections, including parvovirus infection. In either case, exposure may also be followed only by a transient aplasia.

Marrow aplasia may also be seen in patients who have received chemotherapy or radiation therapy (see Chapter 14). The post-therapy biopsy often demonstrates transient marrow aplasia that is usually associated with marrow edema, mild fibrosis, and eosinophilic proteinaceous fluid accumulation in the marrow (Fig. 4.2).

Viruses which have been associated with the development of aplastic anemia include hepatitis C, EBV, influenza, and HIV-1 (Foucar, 2001).

Various diseases may mimic aplastic anemia. Hypocellular acute leukemias and myelodysplastic syndromes may closely resemble AA; difficulties in differential diagnosis are often compounded by the lack of aspirable material for evaluation, a not uncommon occurrence in disorders associated with markedly hypocellular marrows (Nagai et al., 1996; Orazi et al., 1997). In addition, a subset of patients with apparent aplastic anemia will progress to myelodysplasia or acute leukemia (Tooze et al., 1999). The development of myelodysplastic syndromes and acute myeloid leukemia is more frequently observed in patients who received immunosuppressive treatment in conjunction with granulocyte colony-stimulating factor than in patients who received bone marrow transplants (Deeg et al., 1998; Bacigalupo et al., 2000). The identification of an increase in CD34-positive immature cells on bone marrow histology sections can be helpful in the identification

Table 4.1. Causes of various types of aplastic anemia (AA).

Acquired aplastic anemia	Inherited aplastic anemia
Secondary aplastic anemia	Fanconi anemia
Radiation	Dyskeratosis congenita
Drugs and chemicals	Shwachman–Diamond syndrome
Regular effects	Reticular dysgenesis
Cytotoxic agent	Amegakaryocytic thrombocytopenia
Idiosyncratic reactions	Familial aplastic anemias
Chloramphenicol	Preleukemia (monosomy 7, etc.)
Non-steroidal anti-inflammatory drugs	Non-hematologic syndromes
Antiepileptics	(Down, Dubovitz, Seckel)
Gold	
Viruses	
Epstein–Barr virus (infectious mononucleosis)	
Hepatitis (non-A, non-B, non-C hepatitis)	
Parvovirus (transient aplastic crisis, pure red cell aplasia)	
Human immunodeficiency virus (AIDS)	
Immune diseases	
Eosinophilic fasciitis	
Hypoimmunoglobulinemia	
Thymoma and thymic carcinoma	
Graft-versus-host disease in immunodeficiency	
Paroxysmal nocturnal hemoglobinuria	
Pregnancy	
Idiopathic aplastic anemia	

Table 4.2. Grading of severity of aplastic anemia.

Designation	Criteria
Severe aplastic anemia	Peripheral blood: two of three values
	Granulocytes $<0.5 \times 10^9/L$
	Platelets $<20 \times 10^9/L$
	Reticulocytes $<1\%$ (corrected for hematocrit)
	Bone marrow trephine
	Markedly hypocellular: $<25\%$ cellularity
	Moderately hypocellular: 25–50% normal cellularity with $<30\%$ of remaining cells hematopoietic
Very severe aplastic anemia	As above, but granulocytes $<0.2 \times 10^9/L$
	Infection present

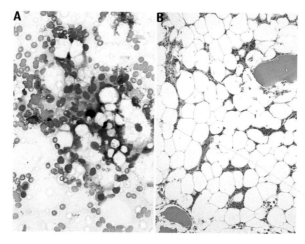

Figure 4.1. (A) Aspirate smear of aplastic anemia and (B) core biopsy. Both show only rare hematopoietic elements and predominantly residual stromal elements (e.g., macrophages) and lymphocytes.

of leukemic and preleukemic conditions (associated with a normal to increased number of blasts) which may be mistaken for AA (Orazi *et al.*, 1997). In most cases of aplastic anemia, the number of CD34-positive cells appears decreased to less than one-third of the normal frequency. By immunohistology, they may appear virtually absent (Orazi *et al.*, 1997), and any increase in CD34-positive cells should raise concern for myelodysplasia. The use of immunohistochemistry in the differential diagnosis of AA is summarized in Table 4.3.

Hairy cell leukemia may occasionally mimic aplastic anemia, but the identification of increased numbers of

Table 4.3. Diagnostic features observed in bone marrow biopsies in patients with aplastic anemia, hypoplastic myelodysplastic syndrome, or hypoplastic acute myeloid leukemia.

	Blast count[a]	CD34 positivity	Megakaryocytes	Reticulin
Aplastic anemia	normal	decreased	very rare/absent	normal
Hypo MDS	normal/increased	normal/increased	present[b], dysplastic	normal/increased
Hypo AML	increased	normal/increased	present, decreased	normal/ increased

Hypo, hypoplastic; MDS, myelodysplastic syndrome; AML, acute myeloid leukemia.

[a] The blast counts performed on the aspirate may be inaccurate due to the fatty nature of the sample, which causes suboptimal hemodiluted aspirate smears.

[b] variable number of megakaryocytes.

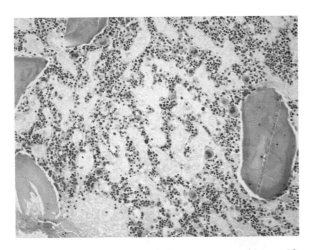

Figure 4.2. Low magnification of a bone marrow core biopsy with proteinaceous edema observed in a patient.

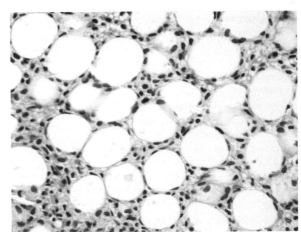

Figure 4.3. Hairy cell leukemia simulating a marrow hypoplasia.

interstitial B lymphocytes in the marrow of hairy cell leukemia excludes aplastic anemia (Fig. 4.3).

Cytogenetic studies are also useful in the differential diagnosis of marrow aplasia versus myelodysplasia to identify cytogenetic abnormalities commonly associated with myelodysplastic syndromes.

Patients with acquired aplastic anemia may, however, develop clonal hematologic disorders during the course of their disease. These include paroxysmal nocturnal hemoglobinuria and myelodysplastic syndrome/acute myeloid leukemia (Tooze *et al.*, 1999).

Constitutional aplastic anemia

Fanconi anemia and Eastern–Dameshek anemia

Fanconi anemia is a rare autosomal recessive disease characterized by congenital abnormalities, progressive pancytopenia, and a predisposition to cancer. The diagnosis is based on finding abnormal, spontaneous chromosome breakage, especially an increase of chromosome breakage in the presence of bi-functional alkylating agents. The peak incidence is between the ages of 5 and 10, and males are affected twice as frequently as females. Constitutional aplastic anemia has two clinical manifestations: with physical abnormalities (Fanconi anemia) and without physical abnormalities (Eastern–Dameshek anemia) (Naeim, 1998).

Fanconi anemia (FA) is considered one of the diseases with cellular defects in the ability to repair DNA damage, which ultimately leads to spontaneous chromosomal breakage (Tischkowitz & Hodgson, 2003). This enhancement is significantly increased in homozygotes when the drugs diepoxybutane and mitomycin C are used. This effect is exploited in diagnostic testing for the disorder.

In the early stages of the disease, the bone marrow may appear normocellular, but eventually it becomes markedly

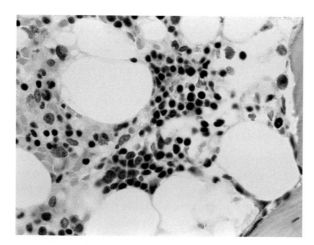

Figure 4.4. Example of Fanconi anemia showing "residual" maturing erythroblasts in an otherwise aplastic/hypoplastic bone marrow.

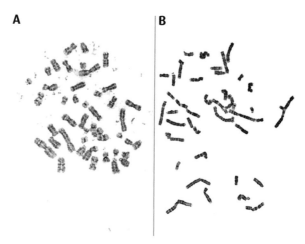

Figure 4.5. Chromosomal breakage study. (A, B) Positive breakage for Fanconi anemia when the culture is stressed with diepoxybutane. (B) A triradial formation is seen in the center with additional breakage.

hypocellular, with erythroid hematopoietic cells predominating (Fig. 4.4). Besides the erythroblasts, plasma cells, lymphocytes, and mast cells can also be observed. In addition, histiocytes may be increased and hemophagocytosis is often prominent in the early stages. The morphologic findings are not pathognomonic for constitutional aplastic anemia and are frequently similar to those observed in cases of acquired aplastic anemia or hemophagocytic syndrome.

Cytogenetic abnormalities, although usually not detected in cases of acquired aplastic anemia, are not uncommonly seen in patients with constitutional anemia. In patients with Fanconi anemia, these include excessive chromosome breaks, premature condensation, sister chromatid exchange, and increased sensitivity of the marrow cells to various chemotherapeutic or genotoxic agents (Foucar, 2001) (Fig. 4.5).

Peripheral blood examination reveals pancytopenia. The anemia is usually normocytic and normochromic, but it may be macrocytic. There may be an increase in the number of fetal hemoglobin-containing red blood cells or in the amount of fetal hemoglobin. Patients with Fanconi anemia may develop marrow aplasia and may also progress to myelodysplasia, often associated with monosomy 7q and acute leukemia (Alter, 1996).

Paroxysmal nocturnal hemoglobinuria

Paroxysmal nocturnal hemoglobinuria (PNH) may be associated with pancytopenia and marrow aplasia similar to

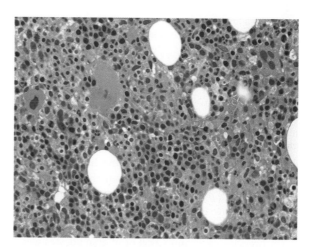

Figure 4.6. Bone marrow biopsy of paroxysmal nocturnal hemoglobinuria (PNH). Note the erythroid predominance and the presence of occasional megakaryocytes.

aplastic anemia, or may result in an erythroid hyperplasia (Parker, 1996) (Fig. 4.6). Paroxysmal nocturnal hemoglobinuria is a chronic hemolytic anemia characterized by recurrent episodes of hematuria that are secondary to intravascular hemolysis. It is a stem cell disorder that is often related to somatic mutation of the X-linked *PIG-A* gene (Takeda *et al.*, 1993). This mutation results in a deficiency of the glycosylphosphatidylinositol-anchoring proteins of decay-accelerating factor (DAF or CD55) and the membrane inhibitor of reactive lysis (MIRL or CD59) on red blood cells, granulocytes, monocytes, and platelets. Loss of

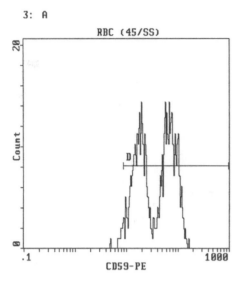

Figure 4.7. An example of CD59 flow cytometry in paroxysmal nocturnal hemoglobinuria. Note the distinctly different populations illustrated by expression of CD59. This indicates that one population has normal expression of CD59 while the other lacks CD59 expression (characteristic of PNH).

these proteins results in the increased sensitivity of the red blood cells to the lytic action of complement. The antigen loss on any of these cell types may be detected by flow cytometric evaluation (Iwamoto *et al.*, 1995).

The presence of positive sucrose hemolysis and acidified serum lysis (Ham test) results have historically been used in confirming this diagnosis. Multi-color flow cytometry methods are now recommended for the quantification of CD59-negative erythrocytes and CD55/CD59-negative leukocytes (Hall *et al.*, 1969) (Fig. 4.7). Flow cytometry of erythrocytes using anti-CD59 or of granulocytes using either anti-CD55 or anti-CD59 provides the most accurate technique for the diagnosis of paroxysmal nocturnal hemoglobinuria; it is clearly more specific, more quantitative, and more sensitive than the tests for PNH that depend upon hemolysis by complement such as the Ham test, the sucrose lysis test, and the complement lysis sensitivity test (Hall *et al.*, 1969; Richards *et al.*, 2000). The defects of PNH may also be present in patients with acute leukemias and myelodysplasia, suggesting an association of PNH with these diseases (Iwanaga *et al.*, 1998). The bone marrow biopsy findings observed in patients with PNH are often similar to those observed in patients with aplastic anemia. However, increased cellularity secondary to pronounced erythroid hyperplasia can be seen in some cases (Naeim, 1998). Stainable iron is characteristically absent.

Red cell aplasia

Aplasia of a single cell line in the bone marrow is less common than the trilineage aplasias. Pure red cell aplasia may be congenital or acquired.

Congenital red cell aplasia

Diamond–Blackfan anemia (DBA) is an autosomal recessive disorder that is often associated with other constitutional abnormalities. Anemia, which becomes apparent shortly after birth, is associated with persistent elevations of hemoglobin F, i antigen, and red blood cell macrocytosis (MCV 110–140 fL) (Krijanovski & Sieff, 1997). Most cases are diagnosed in early infancy (90% by 1 year). Bone marrow examination in these patients shows red cell aplasia with only rare erythroblasts; the other cell lines appear unremarkable. Infants reveal an increased number of lymphoid precursor cells, termed hematogones, which may suggest the possibility of acute lymphoblastic leukemia. Progressive marrow failure with neutropenia and/or thrombocytopenia may develop in a substantial number of DBA patients. The genetic defect is unclear; most cases are sporadic. In familial cases of DBA, a genetic linkage to chromosome 19q13.2 and mutations in *ribosomal protein S19* gene have been documented. Patients with DBA often respond to steroids. Others require bone marrow transplantation. An increased lifetime risk of acute myeloid leukemia and myelodysplasia has been well documented.

Acquired red cell aplasia

Other cases of pure red cell aplasias are secondary to viral infections, drug or toxin exposure, or occur in association with thymoma or CLL (Erslev & Soltan, 1996).

Parvovirus-related erythroblastopenia

Parvovirus, a virus which causes erythema infectiosum (fifth disease) in children, may infect red blood cell precursors, produce erythroblastopenia and cause pure red cell aplasia (Krause *et al.*, 1992; Brown & Young, 1997). Parvovirus-related erythroblastopenia is a self-limited process which can occur in conjunction with a variety of disorders associated with a shortened red blood cell life span such as sickle cell anemia, hereditary spherocytosis, and acquired hemolytic anemia. The aplastic crisis in these patients is usually preceded by an intercurrent infection

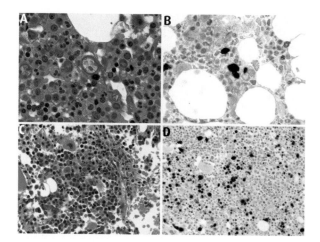

Figure 4.8. Typical findings of parvovirus infection in an immunocompetent individual: (A) an abnormally enlarged erythroid precursor containing nuclear viral inclusions, highlighted by (B) an immunohistochemical stain for parvovirus. Parvovirus in an immunosuppressed patient: (C) numerous erythroid precursors showing intranuclear viral inclusions and (D) an immunohistochemical stain which identifies numerous virally infected erythroid precursors.

such as gastroenteritis, mumps, viral hepatitis, or interstitial pneumonia.

When this infection occurs in "normal" pediatric patients, decreased hemoglobin often goes unnoticed. However, in patients with a shortened red blood cell life span, even a short period of reduced red blood cell production may produce a severe anemia. The virus causes the few residual erythroblasts to enlarge with prominent intranuclear inclusions (Fig. 4.8). The intranuclear viral inclusions may cause peripheral chromatin condensation, so-called lantern cells. The inclusions are usually better appreciated on bone marrow histology sections than on aspirate smears. In the latter, the inclusions may resemble a large nucleolus rather than an actual inclusion (Foucar, 2001). Immunoperoxidase stain for hemoglobin A can be used to highlight the rare residual erythroblasts present in these cases. The presence of parvovirus B19 can be confirmed by staining the inclusions by immunoperoxidase with monoclonal antibodies, PCR (Vandlamudi *et al.*, 1999), or by *in situ* hybridization.

In patients with sickle cell anemia, parvovirus infection has been associated with bone marrow necrosis and systemic embolization of the necrotic bone marrow, which may produce the symptomatology known as acute chest syndrome. Parvovirus infection can also be identified in up to 10% of bone marrow specimens from AIDS patients.

Chronic parvovirus infection has also been reported in rare immunodeficient patients in which erythropoiesis remains active. In these patients, numerous inclusions can be seen in the various stages of erythroid maturation. In immunodeficient patients, parvovirus B19 infection may also cause an infection-associated hemophagocytic syndrome.

Although rare, both agranulocytosis and amegakaryocytosis have been noted in patients with parvovirus infection. This is consistent with the capability of the virus to infect multiple cell lineages. In other patients, an association with immune-mediated thrombocytopenic purpura or neutropenia has been reported. Finally, parvovirus infection has been rarely reported to mimic myelodysplasia (Baurmann *et al.*, 1992). In some of these cases, the peripheral blood smear shows multilineage dysplasia while the bone marrow is hypercellular with dysgranulopoiesis in conjunction with erythroblastopenia. Parvovirus infection usually remits spontaneously; immunodeficient patients, however, may require intravenous immunoglobulin treatment.

Transient erythroblastopenia of childhood

A transient red cell aplasia (transient erythroblastopenia of childhood) has been described in young children (Cherrick *et al.*, 1994; Farhi *et al.*, 1998). A history of presumed viral infections is frequently obtained. Recently, an association with human herpes virus 6 has been reported.

Other causes of acquired pure red cell aplasia

Acquired pure red cell aplasia is not uncommonly associated with medications (e.g., phenytoin). Other cases have been associated with a wide variety of hematologic neoplasms (e.g., large granular lymphocyte disorders), various infections (beside parvovirus), thymoma, and various autoimmune disorders. All causes of red cell aplasia produce similar morphologic features, with the exception of the characteristic nuclear inclusions of parvovirus infection. All demonstrate a marked decrease in red blood cell precursors, with only rare scattered erythroblasts present. In thymoma, suppression of erythropoiesis by activated T-suppressor cells may be responsible for the erythroblastopenic effect at least in some of the patients. In contrast, in systemic lupus erythematosus or rheumatoid arthritis, soluble antibodies to a patient's erythroid progenitor cells can lead to erythroblastopenia.

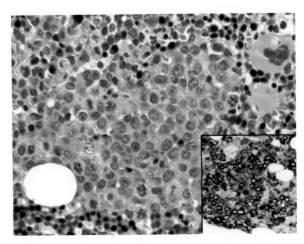

Figure 4.9. Example of "maturation arrest" at the promyelocyte stage in bone marrow. Note the tight clusters of immature myeloid precursor cells with relatively abundant cytoplasm and immature nuclear features. (*Inset*) Myeloperoxidase stain of the same case, showing a strong reactivity characteristically seen in promyelocytes.

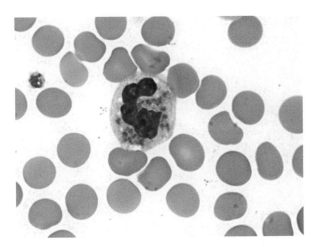

Figure 4.10. A granulocyte in a peripheral blood smear of a patient with Chediak–Higashi syndrome. Note the large abnormal granules in the cytoplasm, which are characteristic of this disease. The abnormal granules can also be seen in other cell lineages including monocytes and lymphocytes.

Granulocyte aplasia

Granulocyte aplasia may be congenital or acquired (Young, 1994; Welte & Boxer, 1997).

Congenital granulocyte aplasia

Congenital causes of granulocytic aplasia include Shwachman–Diamond syndrome, Kostmann syndrome, cyclic neutropenia, Chediak–Higashi syndrome, myelophthisis, Fanconi anemia, and dyskeratosis congenita (Zeidler & Welte, 2002; Zeidler *et al.*, 2003).

In patients with congenital neutropenia due to a myeloid proliferation defect, the granulocytic lineage is severely decreased, with a virtual absence of more mature forms (Zeidler *et al.*, 2003). Maturation arrest at the promyelocyte and myelocyte stages is typically seen in the bone marrow biopsy (Fig. 4.9). The myeloid precursors present appear morphologically normal in most cases. However, in patients with Kostmann syndrome they are often enlarged and sometimes multinucleated, especially the promyelocytes.

In patients with Kostmann syndrome, an increased incidence of acute myeloid leukemia has been reported.

In contrast, in patients with congenital neutropenia due to a myeloid maturation defect, marrow granulopoiesis is increased, but because cells are abnormal, most die within the bone marrow (ineffective myelopoiesis). Myelophthisis

and Chediak–Higashi syndrome belong to this group (Fig. 4.10).

Acquired granulocyte aplasia

Acquired granulocytopenia may be secondary to drugs, infections, hypersplenism, and other diseases. It has also been reported in patients with autoimmune disorders, including those associated with thymoma.

Acquired granulocytopenias are secondary to peripheral destruction or redistribution of granulocytes, and bone marrow examination of these patients may not demonstrate a decrease in granulocytic cells (Jonsson & Buchanan, 1991). Although parvovirus infection is usually associated with pure red cell aplasia, it may also cause chronic neutropenia (McClain *et al.*, 1993). Recently, patients have been reported with persistent parvovirus B19 DNA for more than five years of follow-up.

Megakaryocyte aplasia

Megakaryocyte aplasia is uncommon, and most cases of megakaryocyte-poor thrombocytopenia probably represent an unusual form of myelodysplasia primarily involving that cell lineage (Pearson & McIntosh, 1978; Stoll *et al.*, 1981).

In newborns, megakaryocyte hypoplasia is associated with the TAR (thrombocytopenia with absent radius) syndrome (Hall *et al.*, 1969), X-linked amegakaryocytic thrombocytopenia, or other types of congenital amegakaryocytic thrombocytopenia. In some of these cases, a mutation of *c-Mpl*, the gene coding for the thrombopoietin receptor, has been described (Ballmaier *et al.*, 2001).

Amegakaryocytosis may be a manifestation of either an evolving congenital aplasia (e.g., Fanconi anemia, Shwachman–Diamond syndrome, or dyskeratosis congenita) or of an acquired aplastic anemia in which amegakaryocytosis may occasionally precede the onset of other cytopenias. Other examples of acquired amegakaryocytosis include cases seen in association with viral infections, drug suppression, or immune-mediated defects. Viral infections that have been associated with amegakaryocytosis include measles, varicella, EBV, cytomegalovirus, hepatitis, HIV-1, and parvovirus. Drugs which are known to suppress the megakaryocyte lineage include dichlorothiazide, estrogen, prednisone, and alcohol. Amegakaryocytosis may also be seen in patients with autoimmune diseases and occasionally in patients with lymphoid neoplasms, notably large granular lymphocytic leukemia, as well as in a variety of marrow infiltrative processes.

REFERENCES

Alter, B. P. (1996). Fanconi's anemia and malignancies. *American Journal of Hematology*, **53**, 99–110.

Bacigalupo, A., Brand, R., Oneto, R., *et al.* (2000). Treatment of acquired severe aplastic anemia: bone marrow transplantation compared with immunosuppressive therapy. The European Group for Blood and Marrow Transplantation experience. *Seminars in Hematology*, **37**, 69–80.

Ballmaier, M., Germeshausen, M., Schulze, H., *et al.* (2001). c-mpl mutations are the cause of congenital amegakaryocytic thrombocytopenia. *Blood*, **97**, 139–46.

Baurmann, H., Schwarz, T. F., Oertel, J., Serke, S., Roggendorf, M., & Huhn, D. (1992). Acute parvovirus B19 infection mimicking myelodysplastic syndrome of the bone marrow. *Annals of Hematology*, **64**, 43–5.

Brown, K. E. & Young, N. S. (1997). Parvovirus B19 in human disease. *Annual Review of Medicine*, **48**, 59–67.

Camitta, B. M., Thomas, E. D., Nathan, D. G., *et al.* (1979). A prospective study of androgens and bone marrow transplantation for treatment of severe aplastic anemia. *Blood*, **53**, 504–14.

Cherrick, I., Karaylcin, G., & Lanzkowsky, P. (1994). Transient erythroblastopenia of childhood: prospective study of fifty patients. *American Journal of Pediatric Hematology/Oncology*, **16**, 320–4.

Deeg, H. J., Leisenring, W., Storb, R., *et al.* (1998). Long-term outcome after marrow transplantation for severe aplastic anemia. *Blood*, **91**, 3637–45.

Erslev, A. J. & Soltan, A. (1996). Pure red-cell aplasia: a review. *Blood Reviews*, **10**, 20–8.

Farhi, D. C., Leubbers, E. L., & Rosenthal, N. S. (1998). Bone marrow biopsy findings in childhood anemia: prevalence of transient erythroblastopenia of childhood. *Archives of Pathology and Laboratory Medicine*, **122**, 638–41.

Foucar, K. (2001). Aplastic anemia. In *Bone Marrow Pathology*, 2nd edn. Chicago, IL: ASCP Press, pp. 110–21.

Guinan, E. C. (1997). Clinical aspects of aplastic anemia. *Hematology/Oncology Clinics of North America*, **11**, 1025–44.

Hall, J. G., Levin, J., Kuhn, J. P., Ottenheimer, E. J., van Berkum, K. A., & McKusick, V. A. (1969). Thrombocytopenia with absent radius (TAR). *Medicine*, **49**, 411–39.

Iwamoto, N., Kawaguchi, T., Nagakura, S., *et al.* (1995). Markedly high population of affected reticulocytes negative for decay-accelerating factor and CD59 in paroxysmal nocturnal hemoglobinuria. *Blood*, **85**, 2228–32.

Iwanaga, M., Furukawa, K., Amenomori, T., *et al.* (1998). Paroxysmal nocturnal haemoglobinuria clones in patients with myelodysplastic syndromes. *British Journal of Haematology*, **102**, 465–74.

Jonsson, O. G. & Buchanan, G. R. (1991). Chronic neutropenia during childhood: a 13-year experience in a single institution. *American Journal of Diseases of Children*, **145**, 232–5.

Krause, J. R., Penchansky, L., & Knisely, A. S. (1992). Morphologic diagnosis of parvovirus B19 infection: a cytopathic effect easily recognized in air-dried, formalin-fixed bone marrow smears stained with hematoxylin–eosin or Wright–Giemsa. *Archives of Pathology and Laboratory Medicine*, **116**, 178–80.

Krijanovski, O. I. & Sieff, C. A. (1997). Diamond–Blackfan anemia. *Hematology/Oncology Clinics of North America*, **11**, 1061–77.

McClain, K., Estrov, E., Chen, H., & Mahoney, D. H. Jr. (1993). Chronic neutropenia of childhood: frequent association with parvovirus infection and correlations with bone marrow culture studies. *British Journal of Haematology*, **85**, 57–62.

Naeim, F. (1998). *Pathology of the Bone Marrow*. 2nd edn. Baltimore, MD: Williams & Wilkins.

Nagai, K., Kohno, T., Chen, Y. X., *et al.* (1996). Diagnostic criteria for hypocellular acute leukemia: a clinical entity distinct from overt acute leukemia and myelodysplastic syndrome. *Leukemia Research*, **20**, 563–74.

Orazi, A., Albitar, M., Heerma, N. A., Haskins, S., & Neiman R. S. (1997). Hypoplastic myelodysplastic syndromes can be distinguished from acquired aplastic anemia by CD34 and PCNA immunostaining of bone marrow biopsy specimens. *American Journal of Clinical Pathology*, **107**, 268–74.

Parker, C. J. (1996). Molecular basis of paroxysmal nocturnal hemoglobinuria. *Stem Cells*, **14**, 396–411.

Pearson, H. A. & McIntosh, S. (1978). Neonatal thrombocytopenia. *Clinical Haematology*, **7**, 111–22.

Richards, S. J., Rawstron, A. C., & Hillmen, P. (2000). Application of flow cytometry to the diagnosis of paroxysmal nocturnal hemoglobinuria. *Cytometry*, **42**, 223–33.

Stoll, D. B., Blum, S., Pasquale, D., & Murphy, S. (1981). Thrombocytopenia with decreased megakaryocytes: evaluation and prognosis. *Annuals of Internal Medicine*, **94**, 170–5.

Takeda, J., Miyata, T., Kawagoe, K., *et al.* (1993). Deficiency of the CPI anchor caused by a somatic mutation of the *PIG-A* gene in paroxysmal nocturnal hemoglobinuria. *Cell*, **73**, 703–11.

Tischkowitz, M. D. & Hodgson S. V. (2003). Fanconi anaemia. *Journal of Medical Genetics*, **40**, 1–10.

Tooze, J. A., Marsh, J. C. W., & Gordon-Smith, E. C. (1999). Clonal evolution of aplastic anaemia to myelodysplasia/acute myeloid leukaemia and paroxysmal nocturnal haemoglobinuria. *Leukemia and Lymphoma*, **33**, 231–41.

Vandlamudi, G., Rezuke, W. N., Ross, J. W., *et al.* (1999). The use of monoclonal antibody R92F6 and polymerase chain reaction to confirm the presence of parvovirus B19 in bone marrow specimens of patients with acquired immunodeficiency syndrome. *Archives of Pathology and Laboratory Medicine*, **123**, 768–73.

Welte, K. & Boxer, L. A. (1997). Severe chronic neutropenia: pathophysiology and therapy. *Seminars in Hematology*, **34**, 267–78.

Young, N. S. (1994). Agranulocytosis. *JAMA*, **271**, 935–8.

Young, N. S. (1999). Acquired aplastic anemia. *JAMA*, **282**, 271–8.

Zeidler, C. & Welte, K. (2002). Kostmann syndrome and severe congenital neutropenia. *Seminars in Hematology*, **39**, 82–8.

Zeidler, C., Schwinzer, B., & Welte, K. (2003). Congenital neutropenias. *Review of Clinical Experience in Hematology*, **7**, 72–83.

5

The hyperplasias

Introduction

Non-neoplastic hyperplasias of one or more bone marrow cell lineages are often related to changes occurring outside the marrow and must be correlated with peripheral blood findings, other appropriate laboratory data, and, above all, clinical information. Patients recovering from toxic insults, including chemotherapy and radiation therapy, may demonstrate a transient bone marrow hyperplasia. In a similar fashion, destruction of particular hematopoietic elements outside the marrow, as in some autoimmune diseases, often results in hyperplasia of the corresponding cell lineage in the marrow. Because the bone marrow changes may represent a reaction to events elsewhere in the body, the bone marrow specimen alone is often not diagnostic of the patient's underlying disease process.

Erythroid hyperplasias

Erythroid hyperplasias represent a response to peripheral red blood cell loss or destruction or are related to ineffective erythropoiesis, as seen in some chronic anemias. The causes of erythroid hyperplasias are best addressed in combination with the evaluation of red blood cell features in the peripheral blood (Walters & Abelson, 1996; Peterson & Cornacchia, 1999) (Fig. 5.1). In general, ancillary laboratory testing is needed to precisely characterize the cause of the erythroid hyperplasia. Dyserythropoiesis, particularly mild irregularities of the nuclear contours of erythroid precursors, is common in cases of florid erythroid hyperplasia and should not be over-interpreted as evidence of myelodysplasia.

Erythroid hyperplasias associated with normocytic anemia

Hemorrhage, hemolytic anemia, intrinsic bone marrow disease (including aplastic anemia and malignant neoplasms), and anemia of chronic disease are the most common causes of erythroid hyperplasia associated with normocytic anemia in patients with no history of a toxic insult, chemotherapy, or hemoglobinopathy. After hemorrhage or with hemolytic anemia, the peripheral blood demonstrates an increase in polychromatophilic red blood cells and reticulocytes. In addition, hemolytic anemias may demonstrate microspherocytosis and fragmented red blood cells (schistocytes) in the peripheral blood.

The bone marrow changes seen in cases of normocytic anemia associated with erythroid hyperplasia are similar, and mainly consist of an increase in red blood cell precursors, accompanied by a left shift of these cells due to an increased proportion of pronormoblasts. Such a left shift should not be interpreted as megaloblastic change, which represents an enlargement of both myeloid and erythroid precursors associated with nuclear-cytoplasmic dyssynchrony.

Iron staining of a bone marrow aspirate smear and laboratory iron studies are appropriate in normocytic anemias of unknown cause, because the early stages of iron deficiency may present as a normocytic anemia with erythroid hyperplasia. Combined anemias, such as vitamin B_{12} or folate deficiency coupled with iron deficiency or thalassemia, may also present with normocytic red blood cell indices.

Erythroid hyperplasia associated with macrocytic anemia

Erythroid hyperplasia associated with macrocytic anemia may be related to megaloblastic anemia or to other causes. Megaloblastic anemias are due to deficiencies of vitamin B_{12} or folate and demonstrate peripheral blood changes that include macrocytic anemia and hypersegmentation of neutrophils (Toh *et al.*, 1997; Green, 1999). Pancytopenia may occasionally be observed. Bone marrow examination

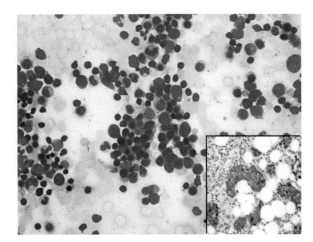

Figure 5.1. Example of an aspirate smear showing erythroid hyperplasia. Note the numerous erythroid precursors in various stages of maturation. (*Inset*) Example of a hemoglobin immunohistochemical stain on bone marrow biopsy.

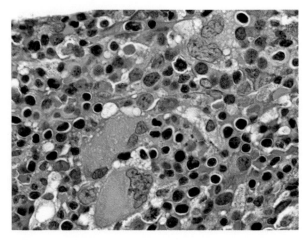

Figure 5.3. Hyperlobulated large megakaryocytes seen in a case of megaloblastic anemia.

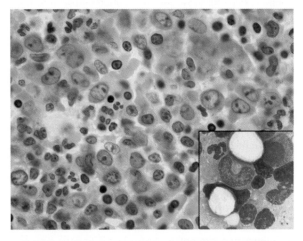

Figure 5.2. A core biopsy of severe megaloblastic anemia. Note the large immature-appearing cells, which are early erythroid precursors. This appearance can explain the historical name associated with this disorder, "pseudoleukemia." (*Inset*) Aspirate smear in megaloblastic anemia, showing a giant band form and a hypersegmented neutrophil.

is not routinely performed for this diagnosis. The bone marrow aspirate characteristically shows a predominance of left-shifted enlarged erythroblasts (megaloblasts), pronormoblasts, and normoblasts with fine nuclear chromatin that may be mistaken for myeloblasts, which accounts for the historical designation of "pseudoleukemia" (Fig. 5.2). Staining with hemoglobin and myeloperoxidase may be useful in confirming the erythroblastic nature of these

"blastoid" cells seen in the biopsy (Fig. 5.1). The erythroid series in the marrow also demonstrates multinucleation and nuclear-cytoplasmic dyssynchrony (nuclear maturation lagging behind cytoplasm). The maturing granulocyte series is also abnormal in megaloblastic anemia with characteristic enlarged or "giant" metamyelocytes and band neutrophils present. Megakaryocytes may show hypersegmentation of nuclei (Fig. 5.3). These features should be correlated with vitamin B_{12} and folate levels since they may be confused with changes seen in myelodysplastic syndromes or acute myeloid leukemia. Cases of severe hemolytic anemia or hemorrhage may also result in a macrocytic anemia with a high reticulocyte count and marked left shift of erythroid precursors in the marrow. In some of these cases, a coexistent folate deficiency may be documented.

Congenital dyserythropoietic anemias

The congenital dyserythropoietic anemias (CDAs) are a group of relatively rare inherited anemias that share in common ineffective erythropoiesis and morphologic abnormalities of mature red blood cells and their precursors (Fig. 5.4). Three major types of CDA and a number of variants have been described. Over the past few years, a more promising breakthrough has been the localization of the genes responsible for CDA I, II, and III (15q15.1–q15.3, 20q11.2, and 15q21–q25, respectively). In CDA type II, incomplete processing of N-linked oligosaccharides leads to a marked reduction of polylactosamines associated with band 3 of the red cell membrane.

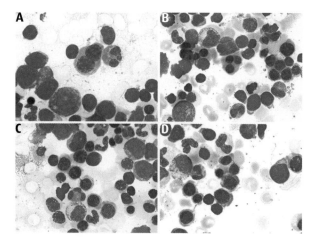

Figure 5.4. Bone marrow aspirate findings in congenital dyserythropoietic anemia (CDA type II). (A–D) Numerous multinucleated erythroid precursors, some showing internuclear bridges.

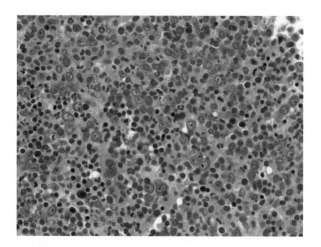

Figure 5.5. Bone marrow biopsy in a case of CDA. Note the marked erythroid hyperplasia.

Congenital dyserythropoietic anemia results in an erythroid hyperplasia (Fig. 5.5), and types I and III are associated with a macrocytic anemia (type II may be normocytic) (Wickramasinghe, 1997). Congenital dyserythropoietic anemia is associated with abnormal bone marrow erythroid cells with intranuclear bridging and varying degrees of multinucleation. The most bizarre multinucleated cells are present in type III, more than one-third binucleated cells in type II, and intranuclear chromatin bridges and less than one-third binucleated cells in type I. Type II is also termed HEMPAS (hereditary erythroblastic multinuclearity with a positive acidified serum test result),

which differs from paroxysmal nocturnal hemoglobinuria by a negative response to the sucrose hemolysis test.

Other disorders may result in erythroid hyperplasia with macrocytic anemia. These include alcohol ingestion, liver disease, cytotoxic drugs, hypothyroidism, pulmonary disease, aplastic anemia, and myelodysplasia. Macrocytic anemias related to these disorders may not have an associated marrow hyperplasia (Wickramasinghe, 1997; Green, 1999).

Erythroid hyperplasia associated with microcytic anemia

Iron deficiency is the most common cause of erythroid hyperplasia associated with microcytic anemia (Meredith & Rosenthal, 1999). Although early iron deficiency may result in a normocytic anemia, untreated patients develop a microcytic anemia with hypochromic red blood cells and prominent anisopoikilocytosis with elliptic or elongated (pencil-like) red blood cells. Thrombocytosis is also often present. Iron staining of bone marrow aspirate material and serum iron or ferritin studies are usually diagnostic of iron deficiency.

Lead toxicity may also result in a similar peripheral blood and bone marrow pattern and may be accompanied by iron deficiency (Griggs, 1964). However, the characteristic coarse basophilic stippling of peripheral red blood cells and bone marrow erythroid cells seen in lead toxicity is not observed in iron deficiency anemia. Thalassemias and hemoglobin E disease and trait also result in a microcytic anemia; however, the peripheral red blood cell count is often normal in thalassemia in comparison to the decrease in the number of red blood cells of iron deficiency (Meredith & Rosenthal, 1999). Some anemias of chronic disease and hereditary sideroblastic anemias also result in a microcytic anemia. Despite the cause, all demonstrate an erythroid hyperplasia in the marrow and cannot be reliably distinguished without iron studies and other appropriate laboratory tests.

Other causes of erythroid hyperplasia

Polycythemia vera and myelodysplastic syndromes are neoplastic conditions that may be confused with non-neoplastic causes of erythroid hyperplasia. Non-neoplastic causes of erythroid hyperplasia must be excluded for a diagnosis of polycythemia vera, and diagnostic criteria are well established for that disorder (see Chapter 9). Mild dyserythropoietic changes in a patient with erythroid hyperplasia should not be used as the sole criterion for a

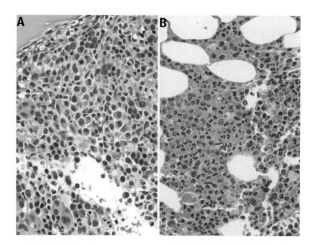

Figure 5.6. (A) Increase in myeloid precursors, including predominantly immature forms seen in association with long-term steroid treatment. (B) Numerous neutrophils seen in a patient with a severe infection.

diagnosis of myelodysplasia, and the exclusion of vitamin B_{12} or folate deficiency is recommended before a diagnosis of myelodysplastic syndrome/refractory anemia type is made. In patients with persistent anemia and only mild dysplastic changes confined to the erythroid series, the detection of a cytogenetic abnormality characteristic of myelodysplasia may be the only means of confirming such a diagnosis.

Granulocytic, monocytic, and lymphocytic hyperplasias

Neutrophilia

Peripheral blood neutrophilia is usually not associated with bone marrow granulocytic hyperplasia, and usually results from demargination of neutrophils or a shift of neutrophils to the blood from other organs. Bone marrow granulocytic hyperplasia is usually a response to an infection, allergic reaction (usually with eosinophilia), toxic events, drug reaction, or occurs in association with neoplasia (Fig. 5.6). The ratio of granulocytes to erythroid precursors may increase and a left shift of the myeloid cells may be observed. With infectious disease, the peripheral blood neutrophils often demonstrate toxic granulation and/or Döhle bodies. In neoplastic conditions, granulocytic hyperplasia of the marrow may not be associated with marrow involvement by the neoplasm (Kitamura *et al.*, 1989). Although organisms, including parasites, may rarely be identifiable in the bone marrow smears or biopsy mate-

rial, the cause of the granulocytic hyperplasia is usually not apparent. An additional cause of neutrophilia is treatment with G-CSF or other myeloid-stimulating cytokines (see later in this chapter).

The primary differential diagnosis of non-neoplastic granulocytic hyperplasia is with chronic myelogenous leukemia (CML) or other chronic myeloproliferative disorders. The absence of splenomegaly, peripheral blood basophilia, and atypical small-sized megakaryocytes in the bone marrow often helps in excluding CML. However, cytogenetic studies for t(9;22) of CML are recommended when the etiology of the hyperplasia is not clear.

Monocytosis

A reactive monocytosis is often a non-specific finding that may be associated with infections, sarcoidosis, collagen–vascular disease, hematologic disorders, and malignant neoplasms (Maldonado & Hanlon, 1965). Among the latter conditions, monocytosis may be seen in patients with Hodgkin lymphoma, non-Hodgkin lymphoma, and carcinomas. Neoplastic monocytes in the peripheral blood of acute myelomonocytic leukemia or chronic myelomonocytic leukemia may have features similar to reactive monocytes, and bone marrow examination is necessary to confirm and classify the leukemic process in those patients.

Eosinophilia

The most common cause of peripheral blood or bone marrow eosinophilia worldwide is parasitic infection, although drugs and allergic reactions are the most common causes in developed countries (Rothenberg, 1998). Eosinophilia can occur with asthma, inflammatory bowel disease, vasculitides, and malignant neoplasms. Within the latter category, eosinophilia may be prominent in patients with colon carcinoma, Hodgkin lymphoma, T-cell lymphomas, and chronic myeloproliferative disorders. Marked dyspoiesis of eosinophils is more commonly seen in clonal rather than in reactive eosinophilia. Clonal eosinophilia is characteristically seen in chronic eosinophilic leukemia/hypereosinophilic syndrome (see Chapter 9), in cases of chronic myeloid and chronic myelomonocytic leukemias with eosinophilia, and in acute myeloid leukemias associated with chromosome 16 abnormalities (Le Beau *et al.*, 1983; Larson *et al.*, 1986; Liu *et al.*, 1995).

A marked degree of leukemia-associated eosinophilia is seen in rare subtypes of acute lymphoblastic leukemias which are associated with the chromosomal translocations t(5;14) (Rubnitz & Look, 1998) and t(8;13) (Xiao *et al.*, 1998).

Basophilia and mast cell hyperplasia

Non-neoplastic peripheral blood and bone marrow basophilia is usually mild and is commonly overshadowed by a more noticeable eosinophilia. It is most commonly associated with allergic or inflammatory conditions, including asthma, allergic rhinitis, nasal polyposis, and atophic dermatitis (Denburg, 1992). Significant increases in basophils, often abnormal, are seen in the peripheral blood and bone marrow of patients with chronic myelogenous leukemia and acute leukemias that are associated with t(9;22) and t(6;9), respectively. The exceptionally rare chronic basophilic leukemia is discussed in Chapter 9.

Elevations of non-neoplastic bone marrow mast cell counts are common in association with chronic lympholiferative disorders in the bone marrow, lymphoplasmacytic lymphoma in particular. These mast cells are evenly dispersed throughout the marrow particles and do not form aggregates or clusters within foci of fibrosis as typically seen with bone marrow involvement by systemic mastocytosis.

The circulating, immature forms of mast cells are essentially indistinguishable from monocytes or may be confused with basophils. As such, increases in peripheral blood mast cells typically go unnoticed.

Lymphocytosis

Reactive lymphocytosis is most commonly related to viral infections, particularly infectious mononucleosis and viral hepatitis, and it may also be seen with bacterial infections. The reactive cells are usually CD8-positive T cells and are large with abundant cytoplasm. In children, a reactive lymphocytosis with cleaved and irregular T-lymphocyte nuclei may be seen with *Bordetella pertussis* infection (Kubic *et al.*, 1991) (Fig. 5.7). Transient T-cell lymphocytosis may also occur with trauma, acute cardiac disease, and epinephrine administration (Thommasen *et al.*, 1986; Teggatz *et al.*, 1987).

B-cell lymphocytosis is less common than T-cell lymphocytosis. Persistent polyclonal B lymphocytosis occurs most frequently in young and middle-aged female patients and is associated with smoking, elevated serum immunoglobulin M, and presence of the HLA-DR7 antigen (Agrawal *et al.*, 1994; Mossafa *et al.*, 1999). The patients have a persistent lymphocytosis, usually between 4×10^9/L and 14×10^9/L, with binucleated peripheral blood lymphocytes (Fig. 5.7). An increased number of lymphocytes in the bone marrow,

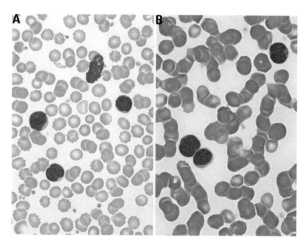

Figure 5.7. (A) Peripheral blood smear showing lymphocytosis characterized by "abnormal" lymphocytes, including cleaved forms, in this case of *B. pertussis* infection. (B) A peripheral blood smear, illustrating findings seen in so-called benign binucleated lymphocytosis, a condition associated with persistent polyclonal B-cell lymphocytosis mostly seen in women who smoke.

bilobate lymphocytes, and nodular lymphoid aggregates may be present. The cells are polyclonal B cells positive for CD19/CD20/CD22 that do not usually express CD5 and are FMC7-positive. The chromosome abnormality i(3q) is reported in a majority of these cases, but the clinical course is benign. Immunoglobulin heavy chain gene rearrangements are not detected in these patients. A role for EBV infection in some of these cases has been suggested. Rare cases of CD5-positive reactive lymphocytosis have also been described (Lush *et al.*, 1991).

Megakaryocytic hyperplasias

Non-neoplastic megakaryocytic hyperplasias are associated with either thrombocytopenia or thrombocytosis. Thrombocytopenia-associated megakaryocytic hyperplasia is usually caused by an autoimmune disorder, particularly idiopathic (or immune) thrombocytopenic purpura (ITP). The bone marrow in these cases shows a normal to increased number of normal-appearing megakaryocytes; however, small, hypolobulated forms may also be present (Fig. 5.8). The overall marrow cellularity in cases of ITP may be decreased. Megakaryocytes with more basophilic and less granular cytoplasm and little or no platelet budding have been described.

"Naked" megakaryocyte nuclei can be observed in ITP, but are more commonly encountered in HIV-positive patients, with ITP-like thrombocytopenia (Fig. 5.9). HIV

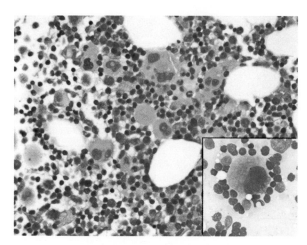

Figure 5.8. Core biopsy in immune thrombocytopenic purpura (ITP), showing increased megakaryocytes. (*Inset*) A megakaryocyte surrounded by small lymphocytes, a feature occasionally seen in ITP.

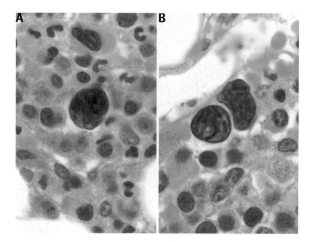

Figure 5.9. (A–B) Examples of "naked" megakaryocyte nuclei. This finding, although not diagnostic, is commonly seen in bone marrows of HIV/AIDS patients.

infection can cause an ITP-like thrombocytopenia as well as other less frequent thrombocytopenic conditions, including thrombotic thrombocytopenic purpura and decreased platelet production due to HIV infection of the megakaryocytes (Foucar, 2001). Direct infection of megakaryocytes by HIV is thought to be responsible for the production of apoptotic nuclei.

Non-neoplastic megakaryocytic hyperplasia associated with thrombocytosis may occur with chronic infections, in the recovery phase of acute infections, with collagen–vascular diseases, with hemolytic anemias, with iron deficiency anemia, and in association with malignant neoplasms. A rebound thrombocytosis may occur after recovery from thrombocytopenia and after splenectomy. Reactive thrombocytosis must be differentiated from the chronic myeloproliferative disorders, particularly essential thrombocythemia. Reactive thrombocytosis rarely demonstrates a platelet count as high as $1000 \times 10^9/L$ and the atypical megakaryocytes of the chronic myeloproliferative disorders are usually not present in reactive conditions. Even when the platelet count exceeds $1000 \times 10^9/L$ in reactive conditions, the number of bone marrow megakaryocytes is less than that usually seen in chronic myeloproliferative disorders with high platelet counts (Buss *et al.*, 1991).

Hyperplasias related to growth factors

Bone marrow and peripheral blood hyperplasias related to growth factor administration is most often secondary to erythropoietin (EPO), granulocyte colony-stimulating factor (G-CSF), or granulocyte–macrophage colony-stimulating factor (GM-CSF) (Schmitz *et al.*, 1994) (see also Chapter 14). Administration of growth factors should always be documented in the clinical information which accompanies bone marrow specimens. The erythroid hyperplasia caused by erythropoietin does not usually cause diagnostic dilemmas. However, some difficulty may be encountered when changes related to G-CSF or GM-CSF are not recognized. These factors usually result in peripheral blood neutrophilia, but leukoerythroblastosis, monocytosis, or eosinophilia may occur. Toxic granulation of neutrophils with Döhle bodies may mimic an infectious leukocytosis. The bone marrow usually demonstrates a granulocyte hyperplasia with a left shift. The marrow morphology may range from a hypocellular marrow with aggregates of left-shifted immature cells with "maturation arrest," mimicking a hypocellular acute leukemia or residual leukemia after therapy, to a hypercellular marrow with granulocytic hyperplasia, mimicking a chronic myeloproliferative disorder (Fig. 5.10). Bone marrow histiocytic hyperplasia has also been reported, particularly after GM-CSF (Wilson *et al.*, 1993).

Although granulocyte maturation occurs over time after growth factor administration, a single marrow specimen may demonstrate a predominance of immature myeloid cells, usually at the promyelocyte and early myelocyte stages of differentiation (Orazi *et al.*, 1992). These findings may suggest a diagnosis of *de novo* or relapsed acute myeloid leukemia. This is particularly problematic in patients following chemotherapy, treated with G-CSF.

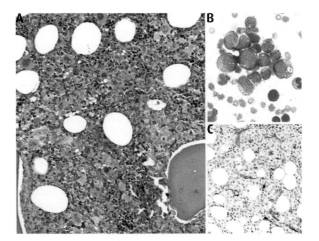

Figure 5.10. (A) Core biopsy and (B) marrow aspirate smear showing changes associated with G-CSF treatment, including an increased number of immature myeloid precursor cells, mostly promyelocytes. (C) CD34 immunostain illustrates the absence of blasts and the predominance of CD34-negative promyelocytes characteristically seen in association with G-CSF treatment.

If biopsied around the time of 0.5×10^9/L WBC, most of these patients will show markedly left-shifted myelopoiesis with sheets and clusters of promyelocytes that may raise questions about acute myeloid leukemia. The promyelocytes in these specimens are usually large with a prominent perinuclear *hof*, do not contain Auer rods, and are not associated with increased numbers of myeloblasts. A predominance of such cells in a specimen should raise the suspicion of G-CSF or GM-CSF therapy. Even when a history of growth factor therapy is known in a patient with a history of AML, the differential diagnosis between relapse and growth factor effect may be difficult. In such cases, immunophenotyping studies to identify an aberrant phenotype characteristic of the patient's original leukemia may help, as may cytogenetic studies. Immunohistology can also be helpful, particularly in cases of leukemia with known expression of CD34 in the blasts. In such cases, if the marrow is "in remission," the number of CD34-positive cells remains unchanged and virtually identical to normal control marrows. In all cytokine-treated cases (including acute lymphoblastic leukemia), immunohistology may be helpful in confirming the promyelocytic nature of a proliferating cell population by showing its characteristic strong expression of myeloperoxidase and other myeloid markers in the absence of CD34, HLA-DR, or lymphoid-associated markers. In rare cases, a follow-up marrow examination after an appropriate interval may be considered to clarify the issue.

The early-acting growth factors such as IL-3 and stem cell factor (c-Kit ligand) can increase the percentage of CD34-positive progenitors/early precursor cells in the bone marrow, an effect that can be documented by staining bone marrow section with CD34 (Orazi *et al.*, 1992, 1995). However the observed effect is modest, with a less than doubling of the normal number of CD34-positive cells in the post-treatment samples. This usually does not cause a problem in the differential diagnosis of "minimal residual acute leukemia." Patients receiving megakaryocytic growth factors are less likely to undergo bone marrow biopsy after therapy, but these agents result in a proliferation of megakaryocyte precursors (Hofmann *et al.*, 1999). IL-11 and thrombopoietin stimulate platelet production by stimulating the proliferation and maturation of megakaryocytic progenitor cells (Orazi *et al.*, 1996). Their thrombopoietic effect can be documented by staining bone marrow megakaryocytes with proliferation-associated markers, or better, by ploidy analysis using flow cytometry.

REFERENCES

Agrawal, S., Matutes, E., Voke, J., Dyer, M. J., Khokhar, T., & Catovsky, D. (1994). Persistent polyclonal B-cell lymphocytosis. *Leukemia Research*, **18**, 791–5.

Buss, D. H., O'Connor, M. L., Woodruff, R. D., Richards, F. 2nd, & Brockschmidt, J. K. (1991). Bone marrow and peripheral blood findings in patients with extreme thrombocytosis. A report of 63 cases. *Archives of Pathology and Laboratory Medicine*, **115**, 475–80.

Denburg, J. A. (1992). Basophil and mast cell lineages in vitro and in vivo. *Blood*, **79**, 846–60.

Foucar, K. (2001). Reactive and neoplastic disorders of megakaryocytes. In *Bone Marrow Pathology*, 2nd edn. Chicago, IL: ASCP Press, pp. 324–47.

Green, R. (1999). Macrocytic and marrow failure anemias. *Laboratory Medicine*, **30**, 595–9.

Griggs, R. C. (1964). Lead poisoning: hematologic aspects. *Progress in Hematology*, **4**, 117–37.

Hofmann, W. K., Ottmann, O. G., & Hoelzer, D. (1999). Megakaryocytic growth factors: is there a new approach for management of thrombocytopenia in patients with malignancies? *Leukemia*, **13**, 14–18.

Kitamura, H., Kodama, F., Odagiri, S., Nagahara, N., Inoue, T., & Kanisawa, M. (1989). Granulocytosis associated with malignant neoplasms: a clinicopathologic study and demonstration of colony-stimulating activity in tumor extracts. *Human Pathology*, **20**, 878–85.

Kubic, V. L., Kubic, P. T., & Brunning, R. D. (1991). The morphologic and immunophenotypic assessment of the lymphocytosis accompanying *Bordetella pertussis* infection. *American Journal of Clinical Pathology*, **95**, 809–15.

Larson, R. A., Williams, S. F., Le Beau, M. M., Bitter, M. A., Vardiman, J. W., & Rowley, J. D. (1986). Acute myelomonocytic leukemia with abnormal eosinophils and inv(16) or t(16;16) has a favorable prognosis. *Blood*, **68**, 1242–9.

Le Beau, M. M, Larson, R. A., Bitter, M. A., Vardiman, J. W., Golomb, H. M., & Rowley, J. D. (1983). Association of an inversion of chromosome 16 and abnormal marrow eosinophils in acute myelomonocytic leukemia. *New England Journal of Medicine*, **309**, 630–6.

Liu, P. P., Hajra, A., Wijmenga, C., & Collins F S. (1995). Molecular pathogenesis of the chromosome 16 inversion in the M4Eo subtype of acute myeloid leukemia. *Blood*, **85**, 2289–302.

Lush, C. J., Vora, A. J., Campbell, A. C., & Wood, J. K. (1991). Polyclonal CD5+ B-lymphocytosis resembling chronic lymphocytic leukemia. *British Journal of Haematology*, **79**, 119–20.

Maldonado, J. E. & Hanlon, D. G. (1965). Monocytosis: a current appraisal. *Mayo Clinic Procedings*, **40**, 248–59.

Meredith, J. L. & Rosenthal, N. S. (1999). Differential diagnosis of microcytic anemias. *Laboratory Medicine*, **30**, 538–42.

Mossafa, H., Malaure, H., Maynadie, M., *et al.* (1999). Persistent polyclonal B lymphocytosis with binucleated lymphocytes: a study of 25 cases. *British Journal of Haematology*, **104**, 486–93.

Orazi, A., Cattoretti, G., Schiro, R., *et al.* (1992). Recombinant human interleukin-3 and recombinant human granulocyte-macrophage colony-stimulating factor administered in vivo after high-dose cyclophosphamide cancer chemotherapy: effect on hematopoiesis and microenvironment in human bone marrow. *Blood*, **79**, 2610–19.

Orazi, A., Gordon, M. S., John, K., Sledge, G. Jr., Neiman, R. S., & Hoffman, R. (1995). In vivo effects of recombinant human stem cell factor treatment: a morphologic and immunohistochemical study of bone marrow biopsies. *American Journal of Clinical Pathology*, **103**, 177–84.

Orazi, A., Cooper, R. J., Tong, J., *et al.* (1996). Effects of recombinant human interleukin-11 (Neumega rhIL-11 growth factor) on megakaryocytopoiesis in human bone marrow. *Experimental Hematology*, **24**, 1289–97.

Peterson, P. & Cornacchia, M. F. (1999). Anemia: pathophysiology, clinical features, and laboratory evaluation. *Laboratory Medicine*, **30**, 463–7.

Rothenberg, M. E. (1998). Eosinophilia. *New England Journal of Medicine*, **338**, 1592–600.

Rubnitz, J. E. & Look, A. T. (1998). Molecular genetics of childhood leukemias. *Journal of Pediatric Hematology/Oncology*, **20**, 1–11.

Schmitz, L. L., McClure, J. S., Litz, C. E., *et al.* (1994). Morphologic and quantitative changes in blood and marrow cells following growth factor therapy. *American Journal of Clinical Pathology*, **101**, 67–75.

Teggatz, J. R., Parkin, J., & Peterson, L. (1987). Transient atypical lymphocytosis in patients with emergency medical conditions. *Archives of Pathology and Laboratory Medicine*, **111**, 712–14.

Thommasen, H. V., Boyko, W. J., Montaner, J. S., Russell, J. A., Johnson, D. R., & Hogg, J. C. (1986). Absolute lymphocytosis associated with no surgical trauma. *American Journal of Clinical Pathology*, **86**, 480–3.

Toh, B. H., van Driel, I. R., & Gleeson, P. A. (1997). Pernicious anemia. *New England Journal of Medicine*, **337**, 1441–8.

Walters, M. C. & Abelson, H. T. (1996). Interpretation of the complete blood count. *Pediatric Clinics of North America*, **43**, 599–622.

Wickramasinghe, S. N. (1997). Dyserythropoiesis and congenital dyserythropoietic anemias. *British Journal of Haematology*, **98**, 785–97.

Wilson, P. A., Ayscue, L. H., Jones, G. R., & Bentley, S. A. (1993). Bone marrow histiocytic proliferation in association with colony-stimulating factory therapy. *American Journal of Clinical Pathology*, **99**, 311–13.

Xiao, S., Nalabolu, S. R., Aster, J. C., *et al.* (1998). FGFR1 is fused with a novel zinc-finger gene, ZNF198, in the t(8;13) leukaemia/lymphoma syndrome. *Nature Genetics*, **18**, 84–7.

6

Other non-neoplastic marrow changes

Fibrosis

Fibrosis of the bone marrow is caused by a reactive (non-clonal) proliferation of fibroblasts which may occur in association with a variety of neoplastic and non-neoplastic conditions (McCarthy, 1985). Fibrosis is usually of the reticulin type, as detected by silver stains, in the early stages, but it may progress to a collagen fibrosis that is detectable by trichrome stains (Fig. 6.1). Normally, reticulin staining is minimal but increases slightly with age (Beckman *et al.*, 1990). Extensive marrow fibrosis is typically associated with a leukoerythroblastic reaction in the peripheral blood that is characterized by the presence of immature granulocytes (usually myelocytes and metamyelocytes), late-stage erythroblasts, and teardrop-shaped red blood cells and enlarged platelets. Diffuse fibrosis usually results in the inability to aspirate the bone marrow. Bone marrow fibrosis is common in chronic myeloproliferative disorders, and extensive fibrosis with peripheral blood leukoerythroblastosis is typical of chronic idiopathic myelofibrosis with myeloid metaplasia. Patchy areas of fibrosis are also seen with bone marrow involvement by mast cell disease (Horny *et al.*, 1985), which may accompany other hematologic malignancies at diagnosis or relapse. Many other neoplasms involving the marrow, including some acute leukemias, malignant lymphomas, and metastatic tumors, result in focal or diffuse marrow fibrosis (Table 6.1).

Marrow fibrosis may also be associated with non-neoplastic conditions, especially inflammatory diseases, reparative changes, or metabolic disorders. Among these reactive cases, a particularly severe degree of fibrosis can be seen in patients with autoimmune conditions (Bass *et al.*, 2001) (Fig. 6.2). Renal osteodystrophy and primary hyperparathyroidism can cause extensive marrow fibrosis, with a relative decrease in normal marrow elements (Fig. 6.3).These changes are associated with evidence of extensive bone remodeling. This includes an increased number of osteoclasts and multinucleated giant cells. Because bone marrow fibrosis is a reactive proliferation of fibroblasts triggered by fibrogenic growth factor production by the neoplastic cells or hormonal changes related to metabolic disease, treatment of the underlying disease process usually resolves the fibrosis.

Therapeutically administered cytokines may also cause marrow fibrosis. This has been observed most commonly after treatment with IL-3 and IFN (Orazi *et al.*, 1992; Heis-Vahidi-Fard *et al.*, 2001). The grading of fibrosis for diagnostic purposes is outlined in Chapter 2 (see Table 2.4).

Necrosis

Conditions associated with marrow necrosis are reviewed in recent articles (Janssens *et al.*, 2000; Paydas *et al.*, 2002) and outlined in Table 6.2. Bone marrow necrosis can occur after chemotherapy for hematopoietic or non-hematopoietic tumors (discussed in Chapter 14). Bone marrow necrosis that is not treatment-related is relatively uncommon. Necrosis may be associated with bone marrow infarction or related to infectious diseases, such as necrotizing granulomas seen in cases of tuberculosis (see Fig. 3.2). Rare causes include thrombotic thrombocytopenic purpura and antiphospholipid antibody syndrome. Zonal areas of necrosis or massive necrosis may be seen in bone marrow of patients with sickle cell crisis.

Neoplastic causes of "spontaneous" (non-therapy-associated) necrosis include hematopoietic malignant neoplasms, such as acute leukemia or high-grade malignant lymphoma (Fig. 6.4), or metastatic tumors. In these cases, large acellular areas of fibrinous, eosinophilic, necrotic material appear bordered by malignant cells. In rare cases, acute leukemia or high-grade lymphoma may

Table 6.1. Conditions associated with bone marrow fibrosis.

Fibrosis associated with malignant neoplasms[a]
   Chronic idiopathic myelofibrosis
   Other chronic myeloproliferative disorders
   Acute megakaryoblastic leukemia
   Other acute myeloid leukemias
   Acute lymphoblastic leukemia
   Hairy cell leukemia
   Mastocytosis
   Malignant lymphoma, particularly of follicular lymphoma
   Hodgkin lymphoma
   Carcinoma
Fibrosis associated with non-neoplastic conditions
   Renal osteodystrophy
   Primary hyperparathyroidism
   Hypoparathyroidism
   Vitamin D deficiency
   Autoimmune myelofibrosis
   Treatment with cytokines (e.g., G-CSF)

[a] Fibrosis may be present in the absence of marrow involvement by Hodgkin lymphoma and may be present without disease after therapy for other neoplasms.

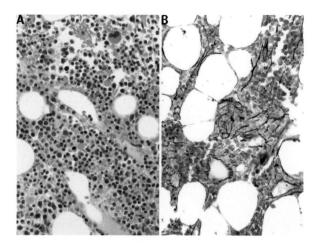

Figure 6.2. Autoimmune myelofibrosis. (A) H&E stain with a relatively normal-appearing bone marrow except for slightly dilated sinuses and increased numbers of lymphocytes and plasma cells. (B) Reticulin fibers seen in autoimmune myelofibrosis in the otherwise unremarkable-appearing marrow.

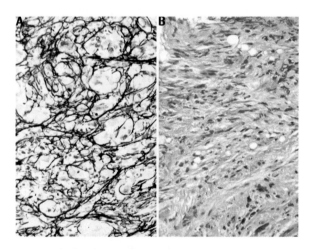

Figure 6.1. Bone marrow fibrosis. (A) Reticulin stain of bone marrow core biopsy showing a marked degree of reticulin fibrosis (3+) and (B) a trichrome stain showing extensive deposition of mature collagen fibers in a case of advanced-stage chronic idiopathic myelofibrosis with osteomyelosclerosis.

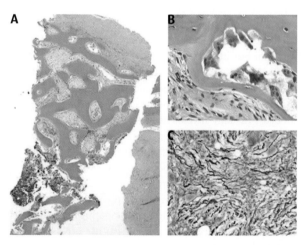

Figure 6.3. Renal osteodystrophy. (A) Low magnification showing subcortical marrow with extensive intertrabecular marrow fibrosis. (B) Increased number of osteoclasts with scalloped and irregular bone trabeculae. (C) A reticulin stain demonstrating extensive reticulin fibrosis.

of the "ghost" cells. With extensive bone marrow necrosis, patients may have bone pain and fever.

Serous fat atrophy

Serous degeneration, also known as serous fat atrophy or gelatinous transformation, is associated with a

present with "total" marrow necrosis. On smears, necrotic cells are smudged, without clear cell borders, and are difficult to classify further. Occasionally, immunohistochemistry may be helpful in recognizing the malignant nature

Table 6.2. Conditions associated with bone marrow necrosis.

Hematologic malignancies
    Acute lymphoblastic leukemia
    Acute myeloid leukemia
    Chronic myelogenous leukemia
    Lymphoblastic lymphoma
    Large cell lymphoma
    Burkitt lymphoma/atypical Burkitt lymphoma
    Multiple myeloma
Metastatic malignancies
Paraneoplastic syndromes with elevated tumor necrosis factor (TNF) activity
Chemotherapy and other toxin exposure (fibrinoid necrosis)
Conditions associated with ischemia
    Sickle cell anemia
    Disseminated intravascular coagulation
    Antiphospholipid syndrome
    Thrombotic thrombocytopenia purpura
    Systemic emboli
    Severe anemia
Infections
    Gram-positive and negative bacteria
    Q fever
    Typhoid fever
    Diphtheria
    Granulomatous infections
    Fungi (e.g., mucormycosis)

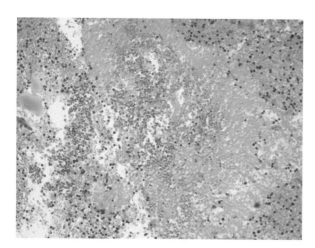

Figure 6.4. Clot section showing extensive bone marrow necrosis, in a case of acute lymphoblastic leukemia. Note that some of the cells appear only partly viable while others are totally necrotic and only their outline can be discerned ("ghost cells").

hypocellular marrow and represents a degeneration of the fatty marrow elements associated with accumulation

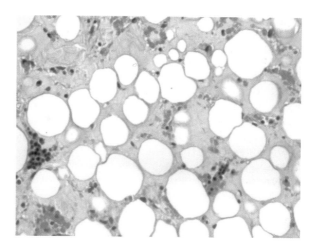

Figure 6.5. Bone marrow serous atrophy, also known as "gelatinous transformation," typically seen in patients with severe malnutrition, eating disorders, and states of severe cachexia.

of extracellular glycosaminoglycans (Seaman *et al.*, 1978; Mehta *et al.*, 1992) (Fig. 6.5). On aspirate material, pink to blue staining material may be seen surrounding fat cells. On the biopsy material, the fat cells are decreased in size and number, and are surrounded by amorphous pink material. Serous fat atrophy is seen with a variety of diseases that are associated with malnutrition and emaciation and reabsorption of body fat, including anorexia nervosa, chronic renal disease, malignant neoplasms, acquired immunodeficiency syndrome, and tuberculosis.

Abnormalities of bone trabeculae

The bone trabeculae should be evaluated in all bone marrow biopsy specimens, even when other abnormalities are apparent in the specimen (Gruber *et al.*, 1981). Thinning of the trabeculae, usually due to osteoporosis, is the most common abnormality identified. Thickened trabeculae may be seen in association with metabolic disorders or neoplasia. The thickened bone of Paget's disease is associated with an increase in both osteoclasts and osteoblasts. The increase in osteoclasts with associated bone resorption and scalloping is seen more commonly in Paget's disease than in chronic idiopathic myelofibrosis with osteosclerosis, another cause of thickened bone trabeculae; however, diffuse myelofibrosis is usually not seen with Paget's disease. Osteosclerotic lesions may also be seen in cases of systemic mastocytosis, multiple myeloma (as part of the POEMS syndrome, see Chapter 12), metastatic carcinoma, renal failure, osteopetrosis, and at fracture sites, including sites of previous marrow biopsy.

REFERENCES

Bass, R. D., Pullarkat, V., Feinstein, D. I., Kaul, A., Winberg, C. D., & Brynes, R. K. (2001). Pathology of autoimmune myelofibrosis: a report of three cases and a review of literature. *American Journal of Clinical Pathology*, **116**, 211–16.

Beckman, E. N. & Brown, A. W. Jr. (1990). Normal reticulin level in iliac bone marrow. *Archives of Pathology and Laboratory Medicine*, **114**, 1241–3.

Gruber, H. E., Stauffer, M. E., Thompson, E. R., & Baylink, D. J. (1981). Diagnosis of bone disease by core biopsies. *Seminars in Hematology*, **18**, 258–78.

Heis-Vahidi-Fard, N., Forebert, E., Eichinger, S., Chott, A., Lechner, K., & Gisslinger, H. (2001). Ineffectiveness of interferon-gamma in the treatment of idiopathic myelofibrosis: a pilot study. *Annals of Hematology*, **80**, 79–82.

Horny, H. P., Parwaresch, M. R., & Lennert, K. (1985). Bone marrow findings in systemic mastocytosis. *Human Pathology*, **16**, 808–14.

Janssens, A. M., Offner, F. C., & Van Hove, W. Z. (2000). Bone marrow necrosis. *Cancer*, **88**, 1769–80.

McCarthy, D. M. (1985). Fibrosis of the bone marrow: content and causes. *British Journal of Haematology*, **59**, 1–7.

Mehta, K., Gascon, P., & Robboy, S. (1992). The gelatinous bone marrow (serous atrophy) in patients with acquired immunodeficiency syndrome: evidence of excess sulfated glycosaminoglycan. *Archives of Pathology and Laboratory Medicine*, **116**, 504–8.

Orazi, A., Cattoretti, G., Schiro, R., *et al.* (1992). Recombinant human interleukin-3 and recombinant human granulocyte–macrophage colony-stimulating factor administered in vivo after high-dose cyclophosphamide cancer chemotherapy: effect on hematopoiesis and microenvironment in human bone marrow. *Blood*, **79**, 2610–19.

Paydas, S., Ergin, M., Baslamisli, F., *et al.* (2002). Bone marrow necrosis: clinicopathologic analysis of 20 cases and review of the literature. *American Journal of Hematology*, **70**, 300–5.

Seaman, J. P., Kjeldsberg, C. R., & Linker, A. (1978). Gelatinous transformation of the bone marrow. *Human Pathology*, **9**, 685–92.

7

Myelodysplastic syndromes

Introduction

Myelodysplastic syndromes (MDS) are a clinically hetero-geneous group of clonal hematopoietic disorders charac-terized by ineffective hematopoiesis associated with dys-plastic changes in one or more marrow lineages together with progressive cytopenias. MDS may occur as primary diseases, or may follow toxic exposures or therapy (Jaffe *et al.*, 2001). Primary MDS is more often seen in elderly patients and frequently progresses to marrow failure, or evolves to acute leukemia, usually myeloid. The overall rate of transformation to acute leukemia depends on the sub-type of MDS, ranging from 10% to over 60%. As a rule, the degree of trilineage dysplasia and percentage of blast cells correlate with the aggressiveness of the disease. It should be stressed that dysplastic features of hematopoietic ele-ments is not unique to MDS and may occur in many reac-tive conditions, such as inflammatory states, HIV infection, endocrine dysfunctions, autoimmune disorders, and may also be associated with certain medications.

MDS have been traditionally subdivided according to the French–American–British (FAB) system (1982) into five major categories, primarily based on the percentage of blast cells in the peripheral blood and bone marrow (Table 7.1), the presence of ringed sideroblasts in the marrow, and the absolute count of monocytes in peripheral blood (Bennett *et al.*, 1982). These subgroups show different rates of pro-gression to acute myeloid leukemia (AML) and overall sur-vival. In particular, refractory anemia and refractory ane-mia with ringed sideroblasts are associated with much longer median survival and a lower incidence of progres-sion to acute leukemia than the other three FAB subtypes and can be considered "low-grade" MDS. However, the FAB classification has severe limitations. Several of the MDS groups are prognostically heterogeneous and a more

comprehensive approach which takes into consideration other parameters (e.g., cytogenetics) has been recently developed by the WHO classification committees (Jaffe *et al.*, 2001) (Table 7.2). The most noticeable change included in the WHO classification is the lower blast cell count of 20% or more for the diagnosis of AML. This lower threshold (a decrease from 30% in the FAB classi-fication) reflects findings of similar outcomes for patients with RAEB-T and patients with AML treated in a similar fashion (Estey *et al.*, 1997, Arber *et al.*, 2003).

The diagnostic work-up of MDS requires morphologic evaluation of peripheral blood, marrow aspirate, bone mar-row biopsy, as well as adequate clinical information and complete blood count results. Correlation with marrow cytogenetics is always recommended (Table 7.3).

The previously used FAB classification was based entirely on findings identifiable by cytological analysis of stained smears of peripheral blood and marrow aspirate. The main criteria for subdividing MDS were the percentage of blasts in the peripheral blood and in bone marrow aspirates, and the identification of dysplastic changes in at least one of the three main marrow cell lines. The new and more com-prehensive approach used by the WHO system stresses the importance of integrating other techniques such as bone marrow biopsy histology, cytogenetics, and molec-ular genetics, which may provide clinically relevant infor-mation. However, not all of these techniques are generally available and/or can provide useful information at the time that initial treatment decisions need to be made.

The value of bone marrow biopsy in this group of disorders is generally well established. It is less known, however, that immunohistochemistry can be used to increase the diagnostic accuracy of bone marrow biopsy (Lambertenghi-Deliliers *et al.*, 1998). This is especially important when marrow fibrosis limits the quality and

Table 7.1. French–American–British (FAB) classification of myelodysplastic syndromes.

Refractory anemia (RA)
Refractory anemia with ringed sideroblasts (RARS)
Refractory anemia with excess blasts (RAEB)
Refractory anemia with excess blasts in transformation (RAEB-T)
Chronic myelomonocytic leukemia (CMML)

Table 7.2. WHO classification of myelodysplastic syndromes.

Refractory anemia (±/− ringed sideroblasts) (RA or RARS)
Refractory cytopenia with multilineage dysplasia (+/− ringed sideroblasts) (RCMD)
Refractory anemia with excess blasts (types 1 and 2) (RAEB-1, RAEB-2)
5q–syndrome
Myelodysplastic syndrome, unclassifiable (MDS,U)

Table 7.3. Common cytogenetic and molecular genetic abnormalities in myelodysplastic syndromes.

Chromosome abnormality	Involved gene(s)
−7	unknown
−5 or del(5)(q13;q33)	unknown
+8	unknown
del(20)(q11;q13)	unknown
del(11q)(q14)	unknown
inv(3)/t(3;3)(q21;q26)	*RPN1/EVI1*
t(3;21)(q26;q22)	*EVI1, EAP*, or *MDS1/AML1*
t(3;5)(q25;q34)	*NPM/MLF1*
Complex karyotype	unknown

quantity of the aspirate sample, producing a serious underestimation of the blast count.

Peripheral blood

MDS patients have significant cytopenias which almost always include anemia, often macrocytic, and an elevation of the red blood cell distribution width. In a proportion of the patients, more often cases of sideroblastic anemia, the red cells demonstrate a dimorphic appearance due to the combination of macrocytes and hypochromic, microcytic erythrocytes. Rare teardrop-shaped cells or nucleated red blood cells can also be seen. Neutropenia is frequently seen and, particularly with the more severe cases, rare

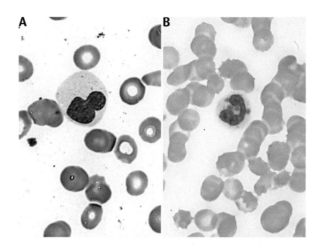

Figure 7.1. Peripheral blood findings in myelodysplastic syndromes (MDS). (A) Hypolobated neutrophils, and (B) an abnormal neutrophil with Chediak–Higashi-like abnormal cytoplasmic granules.

circulating blasts can be detected. Auer rods are exceptionally rare (see later section). The neutrophils often show nuclear hypolobation and cytoplasmic hypogranularity (Fig. 7.1). Cells with abnormal bilobate nuclei in which only a thin strand of nucleoplasm connects the two lobes are termed pseudo-Pelger–Huët cells. Hypersegmentation and pseudo-Chediak–Higashi granules can also be observed (Fig. 7.1). Platelets are often decreased. Loss of platelet granules and giant forms can be observed.

Bone marrow aspirate

The bone marrow is hypercellular in the majority of cases in MDS, but may be normocellular or hypocellular. There is typically a hyperplasia of erythroid elements with an increased proportion of immature cells that show dysplastic changes, including the presence of bilobate or multilobate erythroid precursors and cells with irregular or notched nuclear contours. Siderotic granules and Howell–Jolly bodies (i.e., apoptotic nuclear fragments) may be present in the cytoplasm. The myeloid series may show changes similar to those described in the peripheral blood. In addition, in the more aggressive cases, an increased proportion of myeloblasts is observed. Occasionally it may be difficult to distinguish hypogranular dysplastic promyelocytes from blasts. When these atypical promyelocyte-like forms are the predominant immature element, these cells should be counted as blasts rather than promyelocytes. Megakaryopoiesis may be increased, normal, or decreased. Dysplastic predominantly small-size megakaryocytes are

Table 7.4. Abnormal megakaryocyte features found in MDS.

Micromegakaryocytes	7–15 μm; nonlobated; nuclear/ cytoplasmic asynchrony; intensely eosinophilic cytoplasms
Small, hypolobated variants	
Large, dysplastic megakaryocytes	
Multinucleated megakaryocytes	Disconnected nuclear lobulation
Vacuolated megakaryocytes	

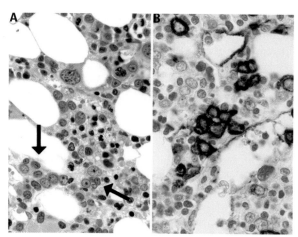

Figure 7.3. (A) Clusters of abnormal localization of immature precursors ("ALIP") (arrows). (B) CD34 immunostain highlighting the presence of an increased number of CD34-positive blasts, often arranged in ALIP-like clusters.

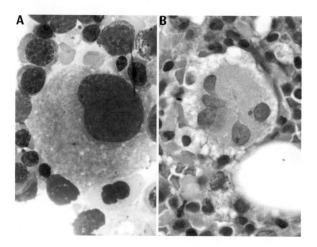

Figure 7.2. Abnormal megakaryocytes seen in MDS. (A) Bone marrow aspirate showing a hypolobated megakaryocyte with immature nuclear features and mature (granulated) cytoplasm. (B) Core biopsy showing a megakaryocyte with abnormally separated nuclear lobes.

commonly observed in patients with MDS (Table 7.4, Fig. 7.2). The most characteristic of these forms is the micromegakaryocyte: a small cell (diameter 7–15 μm) with a single hyperchromatic nonlobated or hypolobated nucleus, and dense hyperchromatic (often eosinophilic on biopsy) cytoplasm. An increased number of lymphocytes, eosinophils, and occasionally monocytes may also be observed.

Bone marrow biopsy

Bone marrow biopsy in MDS allows an accurate assessment of marrow cellularity, predominant cell line(s), presence of fibrosis and/or other stromal changes, dysmegakaryopoiesis (which is more easily detected in histology preparations than in smears), and, finally, architectural disorganization. In normal marrow, granulopoietic precursors are mainly found in the paratrabecular region, while erythroid precursors and megakaryocytes are more or less confined to the central marrow cavities. In MDS, topographical organization is lost, with precursors of different cell lines found in all marrow regions.

Among the alterations detected by bone marrow biopsy, a prognostically important finding is the presence of aggregates or clusters of "abnormally localized" immature myeloid precursor cells (ALIP), i.e., myeloblasts and promyelocytes, in an abnormal central marrow cavity location (Fig. 7.3). Cases are classified as "ALIP-positive" if at least three aggregates (more than five myeloid precursors) or clusters (three to five myeloid precursors) are identified in each section (De Wolf-Peeters *et al.*, 1986). ALIP is mainly present in the aggressive MDS subtypes and is associated with a poor prognosis and an increased incidence of progression to acute leukemia. Presence of ALIP, however, is not unique to MDS and has been reported in reactive hematologic conditions (e.g., status post bone marrow transplantation and post induction chemotherapy). In addition, the identification of the presence of ALIP may be compromised by using paraffin sections of excessive thickness or otherwise suboptimal morphology. CD34, an antigen expressed in progenitor and early precursor marrow cells, can be used as a "surrogate marker" for the presence of ALIP (Orazi *et al.*, 1993a; Soligo *et al.*, 1994). Both an increase in the percentage of CD34-positive cells and a tendency of positive cells to form aggregates have been shown to be reliable predictors of acute leukemic transformation and of poor survival in MDS cases, irrespective of their subtype (Lambertenghi-Deliliers *et al.*, 1998; Baur *et al.*, 2000). This approach can be used to identify patients with MDS undergoing transition to AML, who are therefore candidates for early aggressive therapy. Most of the CD34-positive cells found in MDS morphologically resemble blasts. However, a proportion of the positive cells shows promyelocyte-like cytologic features. These should be counted as blasts rather than promyelocytes for the purpose of blast cell evaluation.

Aberrant expression of CD34 by megakaryocytes in myelodysplastic syndromes has also been reported (Pellegrini *et al.*, 2000). In normal conditions, the CD34-positive phenotype is only found on a small subset of megakaryocyte precursors morphologically identifiable as immature blasts. This suggests that the CD34-positive megakaryocytes seen in MDS represent poorly functional neoplastic megakaryocytes showing, in addition to morphologic atypia, anomalous phenotypic differentiation. However, rare CD34-positive megakaryocytes can also be identified in other types of neoplastic myeloid disorders, as well as in reactive conditions (e.g., megaloblastic anemia).

Immunohistology using vWF (factor VIIIRag), CD42b, or CD61 can be used to confirm the presence of micromegakaryocytes and to distinguish MDS with fibrosis from acute megakaryoblastic leukemia or other leukemic conditions associated with an increased number of megakaryoblasts.

CD117 (c-Kit) has been recently proposed as an additional marker to identify myeloid precursor cells in marrow biopsies of patients with MDS (Petricek *et al.*, 2001). However, in our experience, this antibody is a less reliable marker than CD34, due to its weak and variable expression in myeloblasts. Other antibodies which can be occasionally useful include: anti-hemoglobin or glycophorin A to identify megaloblastic erythroblasts, which can occasionally be confused with myeloid precursors (see Fig. 5.1); myeloperoxidase, which can be useful in differentiating background maturing myeloid precursors, which are strongly myeloperoxidase-positive, from the leukemic myeloblasts, which are characteristically weakly positive or negative in MDS cases; CD68 and CD163, which can be used to identify background monocytes and in ruling out chronic myelomonocytic leukemia (CMML). However CMML marrows often show a predominance of granulocytes with only rare monocytes, with a characteristic difference between bone marrow and peripheral blood findings.

Immunohistologic analysis is especially helpful in three subsets of patients with MDS that may not have suitable marrow aspirate material for analysis: MDS with fibrosis (MDS-f) (Lambertenghi-Deliliers *et al.*, 1991) (Fig. 7.4), therapy-related MDS (t-MDS) (Orazi *et al.*, 1993a), and MDS with hypocellular marrow (MDS-h) (Orazi *et al.*, 1997) (Fig. 7.5). The presence of reticulin fibrosis or fatty changes

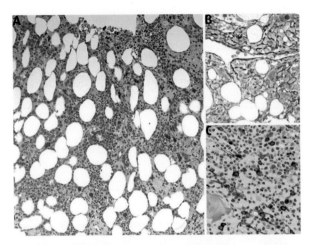

Figure 7.4. (A) Myelodysplastic syndrome with fibrosis: refractory cytopenia with multilineage dysplasia. Note the hypercellularity, the nuclear hypolobulation of both megakaryocytes and granulocytes, and the "streaming effect" due to the presence of fibrosis. (B) shows the presence of extensive reticulin fibrosis, while (C) shows an increased number of CD34-positive blasts without a tendency to form clusters.

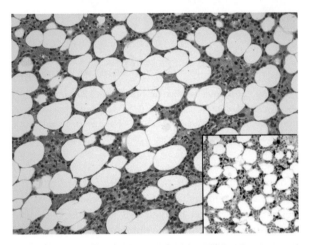

Figure 7.5. Example of a hypoplastic MDS, which shows a poorly cellular marrow. (*Inset*) CD34 stain shows clusters of CD34-positive blasts in this hypoplastic myelodysplastic syndrome. CD34 staining is helpful in distinguishing these cases from aplastic anemia.

in the bone marrow of these MDS patients, by causing hemodilution and poorly cellular smears, can make accurate disease characterization very difficult or impossible. The often-low cellular yield of the bone marrow aspirate may also be insufficient to obtain adequate cytogenetic information, the importance of which has been discussed previously. Besides the presence of fibrosis, other common findings include the presence of areas of edema, increased number of microvessels (which can be demonstrated also by immunostaining with vWF or CD34), frequent plasmacytosis, increased mast cells, macrophages with increased cellular debris and hemosiderin, lymphocytosis, and lymphoid follicles.

Loss of p53 function has a major role in the transformation process in hematologic malignancy. p53 alterations are also frequent in aggressive MDS, particularly in therapy-related cases, and in secondary AML (Orazi *et al.*, 1993b). A proportion of these cases have abnormalities of chromosome band 17p, site of the *TP*53 gene. The p53 gene product can be easily demonstrated in routinely processed bone marrow specimens. In our experience, p53 overexpression is almost always associated with the presence of a complex karyotype and poor prognosis. Therefore p53 analysis of paraffin sections in myeloproliferative disorders and MDS cases can be proposed as a "surrogate marker" for cytogenetics when the latter approach is not available.

It is now well established that solid tumor growth depends on angiogenesis. By immunostaining bone marrow biopsies with CD34 or other endothelium-reactive markers, such as vWF or CD31, microvessel density has also been found to be increased in various leukemic disorders. Results obtained in cases of myelodysplastic syndromes suggest a correlation between increased angiogenesis, aggressive MDS subtypes, and rate of progression to acute leukemia (Pruneri *et al.*, 1999).

Apoptosis by *in situ* end labeling

The rate of cell death due to apoptosis can be evaluated by a non-isotopic *in situ* end-labeling (ISEL) technique applied to paraffin sections (Mundle *et al.*, 1995). Apoptosis assessment may be of interest in evaluating bone marrow biopsies in patients with myelodysplastic syndromes and after cytokine treatment (Raza *et al.*, 1995; Invernizzi *et al.*, 2001). Results from several groups, including ours, suggest that an increased level of intramedullary apoptosis is apparent in patients with MDS, with the highest levels seen in those with aggressive subtypes and therapy-related disorders. In a study of secondary AML and MDS cases, a correlation between a high degree of apoptosis and p53 overexpression in bone marrow cells was also demonstrated (Orazi *et al.*, 1996).

Flow cytometry

In patients with a history of chronic anemia or cytopenias, flow cytometry is most often performed to exclude acute leukemia, marrow involvement with lymphoma, or other neoplastic conditions. When MDS is suspected, flow cytometry is often requested to rule out acute blastic transformation (e.g., AML). In all these cases a comprehensive panel of antibodies, including myeloid, myelomonocytic, and lymphoid antibodies, is generally used.

The traditional flow cytometry approach based on a forward-scatter versus side-scatter (FSC/SSC) gating combination is of limited value, since the only abnormality documented with this technique in MDS cases is a slightly elevated number of CD13- and CD33-positive myeloid cells. However, flow cytometry with the CD45/SSC gating procedure can be used to provide useful information in MDS. The CD45/SSC gating technique allows one to discriminate small populations of immature hematopoietic cells (CD45 dim, low SSC) from the more numerous reactive marrow elements (CD45 bright, high or low SSC). The suspect population can be visually identified by its characteristic clustering seen on histograms. When coupled with the analysis for aberrant antigen expression in myeloid precursors, this approach allows a better discrimination of the leukemic blasts from early non-clonal precursors (Stetler-Stevenson *et al.*, 2001). A relatively frequent aberrant expression pattern observed on blasts in MDS is the co-expression of CD13 and CD7; these markers are normally expressed in less than 0.3% of the marrow precursors (Schlesinger *et al.*, 1996). In recent preliminary reports (Colovai *et al.*, 2002), double staining with CD34 and CD117, markers co-expressed in precursor cells at stem cell/myeloid cell differentiation stage, has revealed an increased frequency of double-positive cells in aggressive MDS subtypes (e.g., RAEB). In our experience, the presence of a decreased expression of myeloperoxidase in CD13- and CD33-positive myeloid cells present within the CD45-dim population is also a common finding in MDS. This finding is consistent with the idea that in MDS the leukemic blasts are poorly differentiated myeloid cells with weak to absent myeloperoxidase.

However, for blast identification and enumeration, bone marrow histology and immunohistochemistry with CD34 seems to be a more reliable method than flow cytometry, being independent of the dilution effect caused by the variable amount of reticulin fibrosis found in a large proportion of the cases of MDS with increased number of blasts. Alternating fatty and hypercellular areas seen in a sizable proportion of MDS cases may also explain the occasionally unsatisfactory cellularity of the flow cytometric sample.

Flow cytometry has also been used to document the expression of the multidrug resistance (*MDR1*) gene, p170, in cases of high-risk MDS (Poulain *et al.*, 2000). Expression of p170 was associated with the presence of an increased number of blasts characterized by CD34 positivity and abnormal karyotypes. However, the prognostic value of *MDR* expression in MDS is still controversial.

Apoptosis evaluation by flow cytometry in MDS

Apoptosis in marrow aspirates obtained from MDS patients can be measured by the propidium iodine staining technique or, more simply, by binding of Annexin V to exposed membrane phosphatidylserine (Merchant *et al.*, 2001). With these techniques a higher degree of apoptosis was observed in MDS compared with myeloproliferative disorders, acute leukemias, and control marrow samples. Proteins that modulate apoptosis include bcl-2, which inhibits apoptosis, and Fas (CD95, also known as APO-1), which induces apoptosis in susceptible cells bound by Fas ligand (FasL). Bcl-2 and CD95 (Fas/APO-1) antigen expression can also be investigated by flow cytometric analysis (DiGiuseppe *et al.*, 1996). A potential prognostic role for apoptosis evaluation is still not established.

Cytogenetic analysis

Cytogenetic analysis, when available, is the most useful ancillary study in the evaluation of MDS (MIC Report, 1998; Pfeilstocker *et al.*, 1999). Cytogenetics allows for an objective confirmation of clonality in cases with subtle morphologic changes such as often seen in patients with refractory anemias. The detection in these cases of a characteristic clonal karyotype abnormality, such as −7, 5q−, 7q−, −5, +8, 20q−, or of complex cytogenetic abnormalities, clearly establishes the diagnosis. The type of cytogenetic abnormality also has prognostic relevance. In the widely used International Prognostic Scoring System (IPSS) for MDS (Table 7.5), risk groups for survival or acute myeloid leukemia evolution are identified by a combination of bone marrow blast cell count, karyotype, and mono- versus pancytopenia (Greenberg *et al.*, 1997). Interphase cytogenetics as detected by the FISH technique is useful to detected "masked" aneuploidy for chromosome 7 in MDS cases (Wyandt *et al.*, 1998). However, it has been recently suggested that the detection of masked monosomy 7 by fluorescence *in situ* hybridization (FISH) may not carry the same prognostic weight as the same abnormality diagnosed by conventional metaphase cytogenetics (Jakovleva *et al.*, 2001).

Table 7.5. International Prognostic Scoring System for myelodysplastic syndromes.

Findings	Score
Percentage of blasts	
<5%	0
5–10%	0.5
11–20%	1.5
21–30%	2.0
Cytogenetic features	
Normal, Y-, 5q-, 20q-	0
All others	0.5
3 or more abnormalities	1.0
Number of cytopenias[a]	
0–1	0.5
2–3	1.0
Prognosis based on score	

Low
 Score 0
 Median survival 5.7 yrs
Intermediate
 (1) Score 0.5–1.0
 Median survival 3.5 yrs
 (2) Score 1.5–2.0
 Median survival 1.2 yrs
High
 Score ≥ 2.5
 Median survival 0.4 yrs

[a] Hgb < 10 g/dL, ANC < 1600, plt < 100K
Adapted from Greenberg *et al.*, 1997

Subtypes of myelodysplastic syndromes

Refractory anemia and refractory anemia with ringed sideroblasts

Refractory anemia (RA) and refractory anemia with ringed sideroblasts (RARS) are associated with a chronic anemia which is often mildly macrocytic or, more often in RARS, dimorphic. Patients are usually over 50 years of age. The marrow aspirate shows erythroid hyperplasia with variable dyserythropoietic changes (Fig. 7.6). Blasts are less than 5% in the marrow and less than 1% in the peripheral blood, by definition (Jaffe *et al.*, 2001). Iron staining usually shows an increased amount of stainable iron. In RARS, by definition, 15% or more of the erythroblasts are ringed sideroblasts, i.e., cells showing 10 or more Prussian-blue-stained large granules ringing around at least one-third of the nucleus.

In the absence of significant dysplasia, ringed sideroblasts, and/or adequate clinical and laboratory

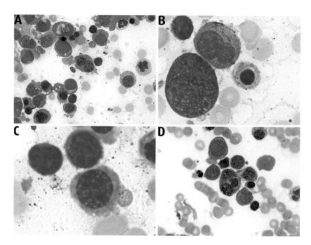

Figure 7.6. Examples of dyserythropoiesis. (A) Multinucleated forms as well as other cytologically abnormal erythroid precursors. (B) An abnormal giant erythroid precursor and a binucleated early basophilic erythroblast. (C, D) Other examples of multinucleation and fragmented erythroblasts.

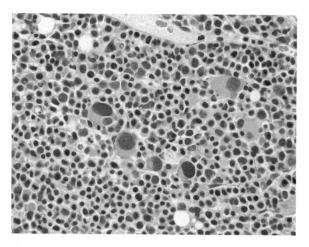

Figure 7.7. Refractory cytopenia with multilineage dysplasia (RCMD). Hypercellular marrow showing left-shifted erythropoiesis, left-shifted granulopoiesis, and severe dysmegakaryopoiesis.

information, a descriptive diagnosis with a request for cytogenetic analysis may be indicated before a definitive analysis of MDS, RA type, can be made. In the absence of clonal cytogenetic abnormalities, the persistence of anemia with exclusion of other causes may be sufficient for an eventual diagnosis of refractory anemia. Patients with RARS but no evidence of granulocyte or megakaryocyte dysplasia are unlikely to progress to refractory anemia with excess of blasts or acute leukemia. Conversely, cases with multilineage dysplasia and/or increased proportion of blasts are best classified as one of the more aggressive subtypes of MDS described later. RA and RARS are the most common and the most indolent of the MDS types, with a median survival of 66–72 months and less than a 10% rate of progression to acute leukemia.

Refractory cytopenia with multilineage dysplasia

Cases of refractory cytopenia with multilineage dysplasia (RCMD) were previously included in the FAB categories of refractory anemia and refractory anemia with ringed sideroblasts (Rosati *et al.*, 1996) (Fig. 7.7). A case of MDS is termed RCMD when it displays dysplastic changes in 10% or more of the cells in two or more myeloid cell lines. If ringed sideroblasts are 15% or more, the case should be termed RCMD with ringed sideroblasts (RCMD-RS).

Separation is warranted since RA and RARS-like cases associated with prominent multilineage (two or more cell lines) dysplasia are characterized by more profound cytopenias and a more aggressive clinical behavior with

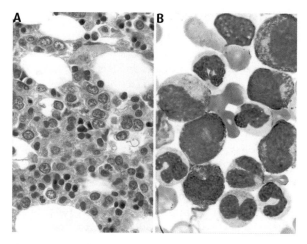

Figure 7.8. Refractory anemia with excess of blasts (RAEB-2). (A) This case shows an increased number of immature myeloid cells, numerous erythroblasts, and several hypolobated "dwarf" megakaryocytes. (B) Blasts and dysgranulopoietic myeloid cells in bone marrow aspirate smear.

a survival rate intermediate (24 months in one study) between the findings in RA/RARS and RAEB (Jaffe *et al.*, 2001).

Refractory anemia with excess of blasts

Refractory anemia with excess of blasts (RAEB) is also associated with multilineage dysplasia and cytopenias but, in addition, presents an increased number of myeloblasts in the bone marrow (Fig. 7.8) and/or peripheral blood. Blast cells represent between 5% and 19% (Greenberg *et al.*, 1997; Jaffe *et al.*, 2001) of the marrow nucleated cells or more than 1% but less than 5% of nucleated cells in the peripheral blood smear. The presence of ringed sideroblasts in the marrow smear does not affect the categorization of a case as RAEB. According to the WHO system, refractory anemia with excess of blasts is further subdivided into types 1 and 2: type 1 includes cases with less than 10% marrow blasts; type 2 includes cases with marrow blasts between 10% and 19%. The latter category also includes cases with less than 10% blasts but with Auer rods present. The significance of the detection of Auer rods with a blast percentage less than 20% in the bone marrow or blood is not completely clear; it is recommended that cases of RAEB with Auer rods be classified as RAEB-2. Patients with RAEB have a ≥25% chance of progression to AML and a median survival of 18 months for RAEB-1 and 10 months for RAEB-2 (Germing *et al.*, 2000; Jaffe *et al.*, 2001).

Refractory anemia with excess of blasts in transformation

The FAB definition of refractory anemia with excess of blasts in transformation (RAEB-T) was based on the identification of 20% or more blasts (but less than 30%) in the bone marrow or the presence of 5% or more blasts in the peripheral blood.

Patients in whom Auer rods were seen in blasts of either peripheral blood or bone marrow were also considered to have RAEB-T in the FAB. MDS cases with Auer rods are considered to represent RAEB-2 in the current WHO classification. Most of the cases formerly diagnosed as RAEB-T (based on ≥20% bone marrow blast cells), are now considered to represent acute myeloid leukemia according to the WHO classification. Patients with ≥5% blasts in the peripheral blood and <20% marrow blasts are now placed in the RAEB-2 group. Previously classified cases of RAEB-T were associated with a 60% rate of progression to AML, and a median survival of 5 months.

5q– syndrome

The 5q– syndrome is a morphologically and clinically distinct subtype of myelodysplastic syndrome primarily seen in older women, with a female–male ratio of 2 : 1. The main features observed in the peripheral blood include moderate macrocytic anemia, slight neutropenia, and normal or occasionally increased platelet counts (Boultwood *et al.*, 1994; Lewis *et al.*, 1995). The bone marrow in most cases shows only mild dyserythropoiesis, absence of dysgranulopoiesis, and presence of an increased number of

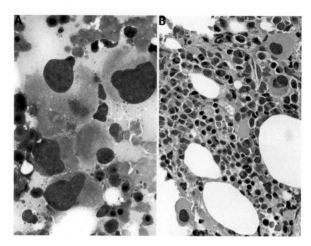

Figure 7.9. Marrow findings in a case of 5q– syndrome. (A) Aspirate smear shows clusters of abnormal megakaryocytes, including characteristic nonlobated. (B) Apparently normal cellularity with increased abnormal megakaryocytes, including small nonlobated and hypolobated forms.

hypolobated and monolobated megakaryocytes (Fig. 7.9). Patients with 5q– syndrome have a relatively favorable prognosis (survival from 28 to 81 months in various series) with a particularly low risk of transformation to acute leukemia, and a low incidence of infections and/or hemorrhagic complications. However, patients with an excess of blasts (5–19%), with ringed sideroblasts (10% of the cases), with multilineage dysplasia, or with cytogenetic abnormalities in addition to 5q– have more aggressive diseases and should not be considered to have the 5q– syndrome. Despite the generally improved overall prognosis of this MDS type, in rare cases, transformation to acute megakaryoblastic leukemia or other AML types has been observed.

Myelodysplastic syndromes with 17p abnormalities

MDS with 17p abnormalities is not included in the WHO classification, but is reported to have distinct morphologic features which include numerous pseudo-Pelger–Huët cells, dysplastic monolobated neutrophils, and neutrophils with vacuolated cytoplasm (Lai *et al.*, 1995). They may occur as primary or therapy-related MDS and are associated with p53 mutations, which are otherwise uncommon, at least in primary MDS (Sugimoto *et al.*, 1993). Since these cases have variable frequencies of blasts, they may fit in different MDS categories; we recommend that both the WHO category and the cytogenetic abnormality be clearly stated in the report. The 17p anomaly is associated with a poor prognosis.

Myelodysplastic syndromes with fibrosis

Myelodysplastic syndrome with fibrosis is an MDS variant (MDS-f) which is characterized by a marked increase in bone marrow reticulin fibers, and which presents with pancytopenia and minimal or absent organomegaly (Pagliuca *et al.*, 1989; Lambertenghi-Deliliers *et al.*, 1991) (Fig. 7.4). The marrow shows trilineage dysplasia with prominent dysmegakaryopoiesis. In most cases an increased number of blasts is seen. The blasts are more easily documented in the marrow biopsy than in the aspirate, the latter being frequently suboptimal due to the presence of myelofibrosis. To qualify a case as MDS-f, a silver-stained reticulin fibrosis score of at least 2+ on the basis of the system proposed by Manoharan *et al.* (1979) should be obtained (see Table 2.4).

MDS-f accounts for 10–15% of primary MDS cases and >50% of therapy-related MDS. Within the subgroup of MDS-f, the classification according to FAB criteria reveals a majority of patients with RAEB. Only rare cases of RA-f have been reported. These rare cases seem to share the poor prognosis associated with the RAEB-f subtypes.

In MDS-f, the presence of increased CD34 expression in the marrow is often observed and the marker can be used to assess the blast count (Orazi *et al.*, 1993a). The use of antibodies reactive with megakaryocytes has shown a higher number of these cells in MDS-f cases than in either normal subjects or patients affected by MDS without fibrosis (Lambertenghi-Deliliers *et al.*, 1991). The megakaryocytes can show a particularly marked degree of pleomorphism with both small dwarf forms and large abnormal cells.

The differential diagnosis of MDS-f includes acute panemyelosis with myelofibrosis (APMF). APMF, previously referred to as acute myelofibrosis, is distinct from MDS-f by its abrupt onset with fever and bone pain. In APMF, histology of the marrow shows marked fibrosis (≥3+) associated with numerous dwarf megakaryocytes, an increased number of blasts, and severe trilineage dysplasia.

Cases of RAEB-2-f, except for the usually less acute clinical presentation, may be indistinguishable from APMF and probably represent the same disorder (Orazi *et al.*, 2005). The differential diagnosis includes also acute megakaryocytic leukemia, which can morphologically overlap with APMF and AML with multilineage dysplasia. Chronic idiopathic myelofibrosis is usually easily distinguished by its characteristic morphologic features (e.g., intravascular hematopoiesis, giant megakaryocytes) and the presence of significant splenomegaly.

Primary MDS patients with fibrosis show an unfavorable prognosis mainly attributable to complications deriving from pancytopenia and continuous transfusions, with a life expectancy of 9.6 months, compared with 17.4 months in MDS without fibrosis (Maschek *et al.*, 1992).

Therapy-related myelodysplastic syndrome

Therapy-related cases of MDS (t-MDS) are usually clinically very aggressive diseases which should be considered as a separate type of MDS (Ellis *et al.*, 1993; Pedersen-Bjergaard *et al.*, 1993). Two main types of therapy-related myelodysplastic syndromes have been described. The first classical type typically occurs late, usually seven or more years after use of alkylating agents and presents as MDS with -7/del7q and/or -5/del5q (Michels *et al.*, 1985; Orazi *et al.*, 1993a). By the FAB system most cases fall within the RAEB category (Orazi *et al.*, 1993a). The second form occurs relatively early, two to three years after the use of agents targeted at topoisomerase II (epipodophyllotoxins, e.g., etoposide, teniposide, doxorubicin), and presents with chromosomal translocations involving bands 11q23 and 21q22, or less frequently other translocations which are more typical of the "*de novo*" leukemias such as t(8;21), t(3;21), inv(16), t(8;16), t(15;17), or t(9;22) (Quesnel *et al.*, 1993). Many of these patients progress directly to AML without a previously documented dysplastic phase. t-MDS with 17p deletions have morphologic features similar to those described before for the "*de novo*" cases with the same cytogenetic abnormality and are similarly characterized by the presence of p53 mutations (Sugimoto *et al.*, 1993; Lai *et al.*, 1995).

The clinical features of t-MDS are similar to those seen in aggressive primary MDS cases except for the more pronounced pancytopenia and anisopoikilocytosis that are usually associated with the former group. Occasional nucleated red blood cells are seen in the peripheral blood. The bone marrow is, on average, less cellular than in the primary cases, and significant reticulin fibrosis (≥2+) is also more common. In spite of the similar degrees of fibrosis in both primary and therapy-related MDS, the latter group differs in terms of the number of megakaryocytes, which are significantly higher in the primary forms (Lambertenghi-Deliliers *et al.*, 1991). CD34 expression is almost always increased in this aggressive MDS subtype (Lambertenghi-Deliliers *et al.*, 1991; Orazi *et al.*, 1993a). In addition, p53 protein overexpression can be frequently observed, particularly in cases associated with prior alkylating agent chemotherapy (Orazi *et al.*, 1993b). p53 expression was found to be associated with increased apoptosis in marrow hematopoietic cells and severe ineffective hematopoiesis (Orazi *et al.*, 1996).

Hypoplastic myelodysplastic syndrome

Hypoplastic myelodysplastic syndrome (h-MDS) accounts for about 15% of the MDS cases, is more frequent in women, and occurs with an age-related frequency which is similar to that seen in primary MDS (Maschek *et al.*, 1993). Previous genotoxic exposure or therapy needs to be excluded since hypocellular marrows can be seen in cases of t-MDS.

h-MDS is generally associated with pronounced cytopenia, a finding which may suggest a diagnosis of acquired aplastic anemia. Bone marrow biopsy is necessary to diagnose this variant. Most investigators consider a case of MDS as hypocellular when the marrow cellularity is less than 30% (Fig. 7.5). However, correction for age is recommended, as a value of 20% may be still within the normal range for patients above 60 years of age (Tuzuner *et al.*, 1995). Within the subgroup of MDS with hypoplastic bone marrow, classification according to FAB criteria reveals a majority of patients with RA (66.7% in one series). The presence of ≥20% myeloblasts in a hypocellular marrow rules out MDS in favor of hypocellular AML. Dysplastic features in hematopoietic cells occur less frequently and are of lower grade in comparison to normo/hypercellular MDS. In our experience, most h-MDS patients with RA have only mild dyserythropoiesis. Since these patients do not have an increased proportion of blasts in the aspirate or ALIP in the bone marrow biopsy, the separation from aplastic anemia may be problematic. This is also compounded by the high proportion of cases showing a mesenchymal reaction, especially an increase of mast cells, and reactive lymphoid follicles, features similar to those observed in bone marrow biopsies obtained from patients with aplastic anemia. The presence of easily identifiable megakaryocytes within an architecturally disorganized marrow and the presence of reticulin fibrosis favor MDS over aplastic anemia.

Immunohistochemistry can help in distinguishing hypoplastic MDS from acquired aplastic anemia (see Table 4.3), the former disorder being characterized by higher CD34 and PCNA expression as compared to aplastic anemia (Orazi *et al.*, 1997). Finally, bone marrow cellularity does not appear to be an important factor on prognosis in MDS, because patients with hypocellular MDS have a similar prognosis to those cases of MDS with normo/hypercellular marrows (Goyal *et al.*, 1999). The distinction from AA, however, is significant because the risk of progression to acute leukemia is much greater in h-MDS (Barrett *et al.*, 2000).

Myelodysplastic syndrome with eosinophilia

Myelodysplastic syndrome with eosinophilia (MDS-Eos) is an uncommon subgroup which accounts for 10% of cases of MDS (Matsushima *et al.*, 1994). MDS-Eos is diagnosed where the percentage of eosinophils in the bone marrow exceeds 5% (Matsushima *et al.*, 2003). Most of the patients present with severe anemia. The bone marrow shows trilineage dysplasia and some morphological abnormalities in the eosinophils, including a disproportion of eosinophilic granules, basophilic granules, ring-shaped nuclei, and vacuolation in the cytoplasm. However, the abnormalities observed are usually less prominent than those encountered in acute myelomonocytic leukemia with eosinophilia (FAB M4Eo). Reticulin fibrosis is usually present in the bone marrow biopsy. Within the subgroup of MDS with eosinophilia, the classification according to FAB criteria reveals a majority of patients with RAEB (50% in one series); RA accounts for most of the remaining cases. Chronic myelomonocytic leukemia, an entity which was formally considered within the spectrum of MDS, can also be associated with eosinophilia.

Most cases of eosinophilic MDS present cytogenetic abnormalities commonly associated with MDS, including 5q−, −7 and +8. Rare cases of myelodysplastic syndromes with hypereosinophilia associated with the presence of dic(1;7) have been reported. In a few of these cases, eosinophil clonal involvement was confirmed by fluorescence *in situ* hybridization (Forrest *et al.*, 1998). Most patients die of marrow failure while about 30% transform to acute leukemia. Cases associated with t(5;12)(q33;p13) and t(10;12)(q24;p13) are currently classified within the myelodysplastic/myeloproliferative category, with most cases fulfilling the criteria for CMML (Golub *et al.*, 1994; Wlodarska *et al.*, 1995).

Pediatric myelodysplastic syndromes and myelodysplastic/myeloproliferative conditions and their differential diagnosis

MDS are relatively unusual in childhood, representing 1–8% of pediatric hematological malignancies, although it has been reported that up to 17% of pediatric AML cases may have a previous myelodysplastic phase. The first systematic attempt at morphological classification of MDS was provided by the French–American–British (FAB) group. However, the FAB classification of MDS is only partially applicable in children. According to the FAB system, the majority of childhood MDS cases fall in the categories of RAEB and RAEB-T (Fig. 7.10). The cases must be differentiated from cases of AML with specific chromosomal abnormalities, such as t(8;21) and inv(16) with low blast counts (Chan *et al.*, 1997). Controversy surrounds the classification of juvenile myelomonocytic leukemia (JMML), which in the FAB system was considered as a childhood variant of CMML. The WHO classification system (1999)

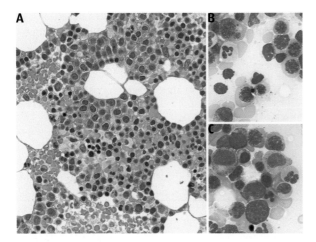

Figure 7.10. Pediatric myelodysplastic syndrome (RCMD type). (A) Relatively hypocellular bone marrow for the age with increased proportion of erythroblasts and left-shifted myeloid forms. (B) and (C) highlight dyserythropoiesis and abnormalities in granulocytes. Cytogenetic evidence of clonality is often required to confirm the diagnosis of MDS in pediatric cases such as this, in which the blast count is only minimally increased.

has separated JMML from the MDS by classifying this disease in a novel group of conditions termed myelodysplastic/myeloproliferative disorders. A proposal for the classification of childhood MDS and related disorders was published by Manabe, 2000 (Table 7.6).

Refractory anemia and refractory anemia with ringed sideroblasts are extremely uncommon in children. Most cases of anemia with increases in ringed sideroblasts are non-clonal. Hereditary, congenital, and acquired sideroblastic anemias may occur (Koc & Harris, 1998). X-linked sideroblastic anemia is the most-studied example of the hereditary sideroblastic anemias. The disease primarily affects males and causes a microcytic hypochromic anemia with ringed sideroblasts which can be confused with an hemoglobinopathy. Many of these patients carry a mutation in the delta-aminolevulinate synthase 2 gene (Fitzsimons & May, 1996).

The most common variants of childhood myelodysplastic/myeloproliferative diseases are represented by JMML and the monosomy 7 syndrome, both disorders typically occurring in young children of less than 4 years of age (Luna-Fineman *et al.*, 1999). Diagnostic criteria for JMML have been proposed by Niemeyer *et al.* (1998). These are outlined in Tables 7.7 and 7.8. Boys are usually more frequently affected than girls. Children often present with pallor, fever, skin manifestations (eczema, xanthoma, and café-au-lait spots), hepatosplenomegaly, variable lymphadenopathy, and hemorrhagic manifestations due to thrombocytopenia. Leukocyte alkaline phosphatase

Table 7.6. Proposed classification of childhood myelodysplastic syndromes (MDS) and related disorders.

I group	MDS/MPD, JMML, CMML
II group	Down syndrome associated diseases: TMD, MDS/AML
III group	MDS
	Refractory cytopenia (<5% of blasts)
	RAEB (5–19% of blasts)
Essential to note related events	
	Post-chemo/radiotherapy
	Post-aplastic anemia
	Presence of bone marrow failure
Minimal diagnostic criteria for MDS	
	(A) Absence of t(8;21), t(15;17), inv(16), t(11;17), and t(8;16)
	(B) At least two of the following:
	(1) Sustained unexplained cytopenia
	(2) Acquired clonal abnormality
	(3) Dysplastic features (preferentially multilineage)
	(4) Increase in blasts

Adapted from Manabe, 2000

MDS, myelodysplastic syndromes; MPD, myeloproliferative disorders; JMML, juvenile myelomonocytic leukemia; CMML, chronic myelomonocytic leukemia; TMD, transient myeloproliferative disorder; AML, acute myeloid leukemia; RAEB, refractory anemia with excess of blasts.

Table 7.7. Clinical and laboratory findings in juvenile myelomonocytic leukemia.

Suggestive clinical findings
  Hepatosplenomegaly
  Lymphadenopathy
  Pallor
  Fever
  Skin rash
Minimal laboratory findings (all three fulfilled)
  Monocytes $>1 \times 10^9$/L
  Marrow blasts <20%
  No Philadelphia chromosome

Table 7.8. Diagnostic criteria for juvenile myelomonocytic leukemia (at least two must be present for definitive diagnosis).

Hemoglobin F increased for age
Myeloid precursors present in the PB smear
WBC $>10 \times 10^9$/L
Clonal cytogenetic abnormality (including monosomy 7)
GM-CSF hypersensitivity of myeloid progenitors in vitro

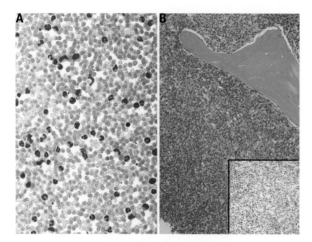

Figure 7.11. Juvenile myelomonocytic leukemia (JMML). (A) Peripheral blood. (B) A hypercellular marrow with an excess of myeloid forms and a relative paucity of megakaryocytes and erythroblasts. (*Inset*) CD34 stain showing increased CD34-positive precursors.

Table 7.9. Juvenile myelomonocytic leukemia versus infection-associated hemophagocytic syndrome in bone marrow.

JMML	IAHS
Hypercellular marrow	Hypocellular marrow
Increased granulopoiesis	Decreased granulopoiesis
M : E = 5 : 1 (average)	histiocytosis
left-shifted myelopoiesis	hematophagocytosis
increased blasts	immature macrophages
Megakaryocytes decreased	Megakaryocytes often increased
Variable reticulin fibrosis	Usually no fibrosis

(LAP) is decreased, fetal hemoglobin is increased (usually between 15% and 50%), and hemoglobin A$_2$ is decreased. The peripheral blood shows leukocytosis with counts of more than 10×10^9/L and monocytosis of more than 1×10^9/L (Fig. 7.11). A variable number of blasts and circulating erythroblasts can be noted. Hypercellularity of marrow (less than in adult-type CML), myeloid hyperplasia, decreased erythropoiesis, dysplastic changes in the myeloid and megakaryocytic lines, moderate reticulin fibrosis, and an increased proportion of myeloblasts are observed in the bone marrow (Fig. 7.11). Immunohistology with CD34 is useful in confirming the increased proportion of CD34-positive blasts, which show a frequent arrangement in cell clusters. A variably increased proportion of monocytes, often better documented by CD68 or CD163 staining, is usually found. CD34 and vWF immunostains show an increased microvascular density similar to what is observed in adult myeloproliferative disorders.

Infantile monosomy 7 syndrome is clinically similar to JMML and probably represents a subgroup of JMML patients. A rare familial childhood monosomy 7 syndrome differs from the sporadic form of monosomy 7 in that, in the familial form, the mean age of presentation is higher and the male : female ratio is 1 : 1.

Cytogenetic abnormalities other than monosomy 7 are not specific for JMML. Similar to adults with chronic myelomonocytic leukemia, *RAS* mutations occur in approximately 20% of the cases of JMML. There is also an association reported between JMML and neurofibromatosis type 1, and mutations of the *NF1* gene have been

reported to occur in up to 15% of cases of JMML without clinical evidence of neurofibromatosis (Side *et al.*, 1998). Abnormalities of the *NF1* gene result in deregulation of the normal *RAS* signaling pathway (Side *et al.*, 1998). The pathogenesis of JMML involves deregulated cytokine signal transduction through the *RAS* signaling pathway, with resultant selective hypersensitivity of JMML cells to granulocyte–macrophage colony-stimulating factor.

Up to one-third of the children who develop MDS have a predisposing genetic disorder such as Down syndrome, Fanconi anemia, Shwachman syndrome, Kostmann disease, or Bloom syndrome. In some of these patients, an association with acquired loss of chromosome 7 is observed. In Down syndrome, acute megakaryoblastic leukemia occurs frequently during the first four years of life and is usually preceded by a period of myelodysplasia, often associated with chromosomal abnormalities including abnormalities of chromosomes 5 and 7.

The differential diagnosis of MDS in children comprises a fairly extensive list of heterogeneous conditions. In particular, parvovirus B19 (Yetgin *et al.*, 2000) and other viral infections, which are usually associated with transient erythroblastopenia of childhood, occasionally mimic the clinical presentation of juvenile myelomonocytic leukemia. EBV and infection-associated hemophagocytic syndrome (see Chapter 3) can also enter the differential diagnosis, particularly in cases in which marrow histiocytosis is not prominent. However, these cases can be distinguished by careful morphologic evaluation of the bone marrow in conjunction with clinical and serologic information (Table 7.9).

REFERENCES

Arber, D. A., Stein, A. S., Carter, N. H., Ikle, D., Forman, S. J., & Slovak, M. L. (2003) Prognostic impact of acute myeloid leukemia classification: importance of detection of recurring cytogenetic abnormalities and multilineage dysplasia on 5-year survival. *American Journal of Clinical Pathology*, **119**, 672–80.

Barrett, J., Saunthararajah, Y., & Molldrem, J. (2000). Myelodysplastic syndrome and aplastic anemia: distinct entities or diseases linked by a common pathophysiology? *Seminars in Hematology*, **37**, 15–29.

Baur, A. S., Meuge-Moraw, C., Schmidt, P. M., Parlier, V., Jotterand, M., & Delacretaz, F. (2000). CD34/QBEND10 immunostaining in bone marrow biopsies: an additional parameter for the diagnosis and classification of myelodysplastic syndromes. *European Journal of Haematology*, **64**, 71–9.

Bennett, J. M., Catovsky, D., Daniel, M. T., *et al.* (1982). Proposals for the classification of the myelodysplastic syndromes. *British Journal of Haematology*, **51**, 189–99.

Boultwood, J., Lewis, S., & Wainscoat, J. S. (1994). The 5q– syndrome. *Blood*, **15**, 3253–60.

Chan, G. C., Wang, W. C., Raimondi, S. C., *et al.* (1997). Myelodysplastic syndrome in children: differentiation from acute myeloid leukemia with a low blast count. *Leukemia*, **11**, 206–11.

Colovai, A. I., Wang, S., & Orazi, A. (2002). Flow cytometric analysis of myelodysplastic syndromes. *Modern Pathology*, **15**, 236A.

De Wolf-Peeters, C., Stessens, R., Desmet, V., Tricot, G., & Verwilghen, R. L. (1986). The histological characterization of ALIP in the myelodysplastic syndromes. *Pathology Research and Practice*, **181**, 402–7.

DiGiuseppe, J. A., LeBeau, P., Augenbraun, J., & Borowitz, M. J. (1996). Multiparameter flow-cytometric analysis of bcl-2 and Fas expression in normal and neoplastic hematopoiesis. *American Journal of Clinical Pathology*, **106**, 345–51.

Ellis, M., Ravid, M., & Lishner, M. (1993). A comparative analysis of alkylating agent and epipodophyllotoxin-related leukemias. *Leukemia and Lymphoma*, **11**, 9–13.

Estey, E., Thall, P., Beran, M., Kantarjian, H., Pierce, S., & Keating, M. (1997). Effect of diagnosis (refractory anemia with excess blasts, refractory anemia with excess blasts in transformation, or acute myeloid leukemia [AML]) on outcome of AML-type chemotherapy. *Blood*, **90**, 2969–77.

Fitzsimons, E. J. & May, A. (1996). The molecular basis of the sideroblastic anemias. *Current Opinion in Hematology*, **3**, 167–72.

Forrest, D. L., Horsman, D. E., Jensen, C. L., *et al.* (1998). Myelodysplastic syndrome with hypereosinophilia and a nonrandom chromosomal abnormality dic(1; 7): confirmation of eosinophil clonal involvement by fluorescence in situ hybridization. *Cancer Genetics and Cytogenetics*, **107**, 65–8.

Germing, U., Gattermann, N., Strupp, C., Aivado, M., & Aul, C. (2000). Validation of the WHO proposals for a new classification of primary myelodysplastic syndromes: a retrospective analysis of 1600 patients. *Leukemia Research*, **24**, 983–92.

Golub, T. R., Barker, G. F., Lovett, M., & Gilliland, D. G. (1994). Fusion of PDGF receptor beta to a novel ets-like gene, tel, in chronic myelomonocytic leukemia with t(5:12) chromosomal translocation. *Cell*, **77**, 307–16.

Goyal, R., Qawi, H., Ali, I., *et al.* (1999). Biologic characteristics of patients with hypocellular myelodysplastic syndromes. *Leukemia Research*, **23**, 357–64.

Greenberg, P., Cox, C., LeBeau, M., *et al.* (1997). International scoring system for evaluating prognosis in myelodysplastic syndromes. *Blood*, **89**, 2079–88.

Invernizzi, R., Pecci, A., Bellotti, L., & Ascari, E. (2001). Expression of p53, bcl-2 and ras oncoproteins and apoptosis levels in acute leukaemias and myelodysplastic syndromes. *Leukemia and Lymphoma*, **42**, 481–9.

Jaffe, E. S., Harris, N. L., Stein, H., & Vardiman, J. W., eds. (2001). *World Health Organization Classification of Tumours: Pathology and Genetics of Tumours of Haematopoietic and Lymphoid Tissues*. Lyon: IARC Press.

Jakovleva, K., Ogard, I., Arvidsson, I., Jacobsson, B., Swolin, B., & Hast, R. (2001). Masked monosomy 7 in myelodysplastic syndromes is uncommon and of undetermined clinical significance. *Leukemia Research*, **25**, 197–203.

Koc, S. & Harris, J. W. (1998). Sideroblastic anemias: variations of imprecision in diagnostic criteria, proposal for an extended classification of sideroblastic anemias. *American Journal of Hematology*, **57**, 1–6.

Lai, J. L., Preudhomme, C., Zandecki, M., *et al.* (1995). Myelodysplastic syndromes and acute myeloid leukemia with 17-p deletion: an entity characterized by specific dysgranulopoiesis and a high incidence of p53 mutations. *Leukemia*, **9**, 370–81.

Lambertenghi-Deliliers, G., Orazi, A., Luksch, R., Annaloro, C., & Soligo, D. (1991). Myelodysplastic syndrome with increased marrow fibrosis: a distinct clinico-pathological entity. *British Journal of Haematology*, **78**, 161–6.

Lambertenghi-Deliliers, G., Annaloro, C., Soligo, D., & Oriani, A. (1998). The diagnostic and prognostic value of bone marrow immunostaining in myelodysplastic syndromes. *Leukemia and Lymphoma*, **28**, 231–9.

Lewis, S., Oscier, D., Boultwood, J., *et al.* (1995). Hematological features of patients with myelodysplastic syndromes associated with a chromosome 5q deletion. *American Journal of Hematology*, **49**, 194–200.

Luna-Fineman, S., Shannon, K. M., Atwater, S. K., *et al.* (1999). Myelodysplastic and myeloproliferative disorders of childhood: a study of 167 patients. *Blood*, **93**, 459–66.

Manabe, A. (2000). Second international symposium on myelodysplastic syndromes in childhood. *International Journal of Hematology*, **72**, 522–4.

Manoharan, A., Horsley, R., & Pitney, W. R. (1979). The reticulin content of bone marrow in acute leukaemia in adults. *British Journal of Haematology*, **43**, 185–90.

Maschek, H., Georgii, A., Kaloutski, V., *et al.* (1992). Myelofibrosis in primary myelodysplastic syndromes: a retrospective study of 352 patients. *European Journal of Haematology*, **48**, 208–14.

Maschek, H., Kaloutsi, V., Rodriguez-Kaiser, M., *et al.* (1993). Hypoplastic myelodysplastic syndrome: incidence, morphology, cytogenetics, and prognosis. *Annals of Hematopathology*, **66**, 117–22.

Matsushima, T., Murakami, H., & Tsuchiya, J. (1994). Myelodysplastic syndrome with bone marrow eosinophilia: clinical and cytogenetic features. *Leukemia and Lymphoma*, **15**, 491–7.

Matsushima, T., Handa, H., Yokohama, A., *et al.* (2003). Prevalence and clinical characteristics of myelodysplastic syndrome with bone marrow eosinophilia or basophilia. *Blood*, **101**, 3386–90.

Merchant, S. H., Gonchoroff, N. J., & Hutchison, R. E. (2001). Apoptotic index by Annexin V flow cytometry: adjunct to morphologic and cytogenetic diagnosis of myelodysplastic syndromes. *Cytometry*, **46**, 28–32.

MIC Report (1998). Recommendations for a morphologic, immunologic, and cytogenetic (MIC) working classification of the primary and therapy-related myelodysplastic disorders: report of the workshop held in Scottsdale, Arizona, USA, on February 23–25, 1987. Third MIC Cooperative Study Group. *Cancer Genetics and Cytogenetics*, **32**, 1–10.

Michels, S. D., McKenna, R. W., Arthur, D.C., & Brunning, R. D. (1985). Therapy-related acute myeloid leukemia and myelodysplastic syndrome: a clinical and morphologic study of 65 cases. *Blood*, **65**, 1364–72.

Mundle, S. D., Gao, X. Z., Khan, S., Gregory, S. A., Preisler, H. D., & Raza, A. (1995). Two in situ labeling techniques reveal different patterns of DNA fragmentation during spontaneous apoptosis in vivo and induced apoptosis in vitro. *Anticancer Research*, **15**, 1895–904.

Niemeyer, C. M., Fenu, S., Hasle, H., Mann, G., Stary, J., & van Wering, E. (1998). Response: differentiating juvenile myelomonocytic leukemia from infectious disease. *Blood*, **91**, 365–6.

Orazi, A., Cattoretti, G., Soligo, D., Luksch, R., & Lambertenghi-Deliliers, G. (1993a). Therapy-related myelodysplastic syndromes: FAB classification, bone marrow histology, and immunohistology in the prognostic assessment. *Leukemia*, **7**, 838–47.

Orazi, A., Cattoretti, G., Heerema, N. A., Sozzi, G., John, K., & Neiman, R. S. (1993b). Frequent p53 overexpression in therapy related myelodysplastic syndromes and acute myeloid leukemias: an immunohistochemical study of bone marrow biopsies. *Modern Pathology*, **6**, 521–5.

Orazi, A., Kahsai, M., John, K., & Neiman, R. S. (1996). p53 overexpression in myeloid leukemic disorders is associated with increased apoptosis of hematopoietic marrow cells and ineffective hematopoiesis. *Modern Pathology*, **9**, 48–52.

Orazi, A., Albitar, M., Heerema, N. A., Haskins, S., & Neiman, R. S. (1997). Hypoplastic myelodysplastic syndromes can be distinguished from acquired aplastic anemia by CD34 and PCNA immunostaining of bone marrow biopsy specimens. *American Journal of Clinical Pathology*, **107**, 268–74.

Orazi, A., O'Malley, D. P., Jiang, J., *et al.* (2005). Acute panmyelosis with myelofibrosis: an entity distinct from acute megakaryoblastic leukemia. *Modern Pathology*, **18**, 603–14.

Pagliuca, A., Layton, D. M., Manoharan, A., Gordon, S., Green, P. J., & Mufti, G. J. (1989). Myelofibrosis in primary myelodysplastic syndromes: a clinico-morphological study of 10 cases. *British Journal of Haematology*, **71**, 499–504.

Pedersen-Bjergaard, J., Philip, P., Larsen, S. O., *et al.* (1993). Therapy-related myelodysplasia and acute myeloid leukemia: cytogenetic characteristics of 115 consecutive cases and risk in seven cohorts of patients treated intensively for malignant diseases in the Copenhagen series. *Leukemia*, **7**, 1975–86.

Pellegrini, W., Facchetti, F., Marocolo, D., Pelizzari, A. M., Capucci, A., & Rossi, G. (2000). Expression of CD34 by megakaryocytes in myelodysplastic syndromes. *Haematologica*, **85**, 1117–18.

Petricek, C. M., Ross, C. W., Finn, W. G., Schnitzer, B., & Singleton, T. P. (2001). Utility of anti-CD117 in the flow cytometric analysis of acute leukemia. *Modern Pathology*, **13**, 160A.

Pfeilstocker, M., Reisner, R., Nosslinger, T., *et al.* (1999). Cross-validations of prognostic scores in myelodysplastic syndromes on 386 patients from a single institution confirm importance of cytogenetics. *British Journal of Haematology*, **106**, 455–63.

Poulain, S., Lepelley, P., Preudhomme, C., *et al.* (2000). Expression of the multidrug resistance-associated protein in myelodysplastic syndromes. *British Journal of Haematology*, **110**, 591–8.

Pruneri, G., Bertolini, F., Soligo, D., *et al.* (1999). Angiogenesis in myelodysplastic syndromes. *British Journal of Cancer*, **81**, 1398–401.

Quesnel, B., Kantarjian, H., Bjergaard, J. P., *et al.* (1993). Therapy-related acute myeloid leukemia with t(8;21), inv(16), and t(8;16): a report on 25 cases and review of the literature. *Journal of Clinical Oncology*, **11**, 2370–9.

Raza, A., Gezer, S., Mundle, S., *et al.* (1995). Apoptosis in bone marrow biopsy samples involving stromal and hematopoietic cells in 50 patients with myelodysplastic syndromes. *Blood*, **86**, 268–76.

Rosati, S., Mick, R., Xu, F., *et al.* (1996). Refractory cytopenia with multilineage dysplasia: further characterization of an "unclassifiable" myelodysplastic syndrome. *Leukemia*, **10**, 20–6.

Schlesinger, M., Silverman, L. R., Jiang, J. D., Yagi, M. J., Holland, J. F., & Bekesi, J. G. (1996). Analysis of myeloid and lymphoid markers on the surface and in the cytoplasm of mononuclear bone marrow cells in patients with myelodysplastic syndrome. *Journal of Clinical and Laboratory Immunology*, **48**, 149–66.

Side, L. E, Emanuel, P. D., Taylor, B., *et al.* (1998). Mutations of the NF1 gene in children with juvenile myelomonocytic leukemia without clinical evidence of neurofibromatosis, type 1. *Blood*, **92**, 267–72.

Soligo, D. A., Oriani, A., Annaloro, C., *et al.* (1994). CD34 immunohistochemistry of bone marrow biopsies: prognostic significance in primary myelodysplastic syndromes. *American Journal of Hematology*, **46**, 9–17.

Stetler-Stevenson, M., Arthur, D.C., Jabbour, N., *et al.* (2001). Diagnostic utility of flow cytometric immunophenotyping in myelodysplastic syndrome. *Blood*, **98**, 979–87.

Sugimoto, K., Hirano, N., Toyoshima, H., *et al.* (1993). Mutations of the p53 gene in myelodysplastic syndrome (MDS) and MDS-derived leukemia. *Blood*, **81**, 3022–6.

Tuzuner, N., Cox, C., Rowe, J. M., Watrous, D., & Bennett, J. M. (1995). Hypocellular myelodysplastic syndromes (MDS): new proposals. *British Journal of Haematology*, **91**, 612–17.

Wlodarska, I., Mecucci, C., Marynen, P., *et al.* (1995). TEL gene is involved in myelodysplastic syndromes with either the typical t(5;12)(q33;p13) translocation or its variant t(10;12)(q24;p13). *Blood*, **85**, 2848–52.

Wyandt, H. E., Chinnappan, D., Ioannidou, S., Salama, M., & O'Hara, C. (1998). Fluorescence in situ hybridization to assess aneuploidy for chromosomes 7 and 8 in hematologic disorders. *Cancer Genetics and Cytogenetics*, **102**, 114–24.

Yetgin, S., Cetin, M., Yenicesu, I., Ozaltin, F., & Uckan, D. (2000). Acute parvovirus B19 infection mimicking juvenile myelomonocytic leukemia. *European Journal of Haematology*, **65**, 276–8.

8

Acute leukemia

Introduction

Acute leukemia is a proliferation of immature bone marrow-derived cells (blasts) that may also involve peripheral blood or solid organs. The percentage of bone marrow blast cells required for a diagnosis of acute leukemia has traditionally been set arbitrarily at 30% or more. However, more recently proposed classification systems have lowered the blast cell count to 20% for many leukemia types, and do not require any minimum blast cell percentage when certain morphologic and cytogenetic features are present.

The traditional classification of acute leukemia used criteria proposed by the French–American–British Cooperative Group (FAB) (Table 8.1), using the 30% bone marrow blast cell cutoff (Bennett *et al.*, 1976, 1985a). This classification system originally distinguished different leukemia types by morphologic features and cytochemical studies, particularly myeloperoxidase (or Sudan black B) and non-specific esterase staining. It was revised to include leukemia types that could only be accurately identified with the addition of immunophenotyping or electron microscopic studies (Bennett *et al.*, 1985b, 1991). Although the FAB classification failed to distinguish immunophenotypic groups of acute lymphoblastic leukemias, did not recognize the significance of myelodysplastic changes in acute myeloid leukemias or cytogenetic abnormalities in either leukemia type, and resulted in some subcategories of little clinical significance, this system provided very clear guidelines for classification. In addition, some distinct leukemia subtypes, particularly acute promyelocytic leukemia and acute myeloid leukemia with abnormal eosinophils, were found to correlate with specific cytogenetic aberrations and had unique clinical features, and those remain in recently proposed classification systems.

The significance of cytogenetic abnormalities in acute leukemia and of associated myelodysplasia in acute myeloid leukemia has become apparent since the introduction of the FAB classification, and more recently proposed systems have attempted to incorporate these factors. The World Health Organization Classification of Neoplastic Diseases of the Hematopoietic and Lymphoid Tissues (WHO classification) (Harris *et al.*, 1999; Jaffe *et al.*, 2001), which includes acute leukemia (Table 8.2), and the Realistic Pathologic Classification of acute myeloid leukemia (Arber, 2001; Arber *et al.*, 2003a) (Table 8.3) have both attempted to recognize distinct subgroups of acute leukemia that were not included in the FAB classification. Both of these systems lower the required blast cell count for most diseases to 20% for a diagnosis of acute leukemia, essentially eliminating a diagnosis of refractory anemia with excess blasts in transformation, and have no blast cell requirement for acute myeloid leukemias with recurring cytogenetic translocations. The WHO classification, which also includes acute lymphoblastic leukemia (ALL), requires immunophenotyping to identify ALL types, and the detection of immunophenotypic abnormalities specific for certain acute leukemia subtypes can be helpful in the classification of these diseases. While flow cytometry immunophenotyping is preferred, paraffin section immunohistochemistry can be useful when aspirate material is not available (Arber & Jenkins, 1996; Manaloor *et al.*, 2000).

Therefore, the diagnosis and subclassification of acute leukemia now requires a combination of morphology, cytochemistry, immunophenotyping, and cytogenetics (or molecular genetics) for complete diagnosis of many of the disease types. The most common balanced cytogenetic abnormalities in acute leukemia are listed in Table 8.4. This chapter will summarize the features of the major disease types of all three classification systems. Although adult

Table 8.1. French–American–British Cooperative Group (FAB) classification of acute leukemia.

Acute myeloid leukemia
M0	Minimally differentiated acute myeloid leukemia
M1	Myeloblastic leukemia without maturation
M2	Myeloblastic leukemia with maturation
M3	Promyelocytic leukemia
M3v	Microgranular variant, promyelocytic leukemia
M4	Myelomonocytic leukemia
M4Eo	Myelomonocytic leukemia with eosinophils
M5a	Monoblastic leukemia (poorly differentiated)
M5b	Monocytic leukemia (differentiated)
M6	Erythroleukemia
M7	Megakaryoblastic leukemia

Acute lymphoblastic leukemia
L1	
L2	
L3 (Burkitt)	

and pediatric leukemia will be presented together, there are marked differences in the incidence and prognosis of certain disease types by age, and these differences will be highlighted.

Acute lymphoblastic leukemia

The FAB classification separates acute lymphoblastic leukemia (ALL) into three morphologic types, L1, L2, and L3 (Bennett *et al.*, 1981) (Fig. 8.1). L1 blasts have fine nuclear chromatin with small, indistinct nucleoli, fairly uniformly sized nuclei, and scant, agranular cytoplasm. L2 blasts are heterogeneous, with more variation in nuclear size, and may have more prominent nucleoli and more abundant cytoplasm. L3 blasts have more mature nuclei, with chromatin clumping and multiple distinct nucleoli, deeply basophilic cytoplasm, and prominent cytoplasmic vacuoles. L2 morphology in children may be associated with a worse prognosis, but this is probably related more to cytogenetic abnormalities than to blast cell morphology alone. L1 and L2 blast morphology tends to correlate with a precursor lymphoid immunophenotype, while L3 morphology is more characteristic of a mature B-cell immunophenotype. L1 and L2 blasts may be seen in both the precursor B-cell and precursor T-cell subtypes of the WHO classification, and there is probably little if any significance in separating blast cells into the L1 and L2 groups.

The WHO classification separates ALL into precursor B-cell and precursor T-cell types of ALL, which are felt to represent leukemic presentation related to the lymphoblastic

Table 8.2. World Health Organization (WHO) classification categories of acute leukemia.

Lymphoid neoplasms
Precursor B lymphoblastic leukemia/lymphoblastic lymphoma
Precursor T lymphoblastic leukemia/lymphoblastic lymphoma
Burkitt lymphoma/leukemia

Acute myeloid leukemias
Acute myeloid leukemia with recurrent cytogenetic translocations
Acute myeloid leukemia with t(8;21)(q22;q22);
   (AML1(CBFα)/ETO)
Acute myeloid leukemia with abnormal bone marrow
   eosinophils inv(16)(p13q22) or t(16;16)(p13;q22);
   (CBFβ/MYH11)
Acute promyelocytic leukemia (AML) with t(15;17)(q22;q112);
   (PML/RARα) and variants
Acute myeloid leukemia with 11q23 (MLL) abnormalities
Acute myeloid leukemia with multilineage dysplasia
Acute myeloid leukemia and myelodysplastic syndromes,
   therapy-related
Acute myeloid leukemia not otherwise categorized
Acute myeloid leukemia minimally differentiated
Acute myeloid leukemia without maturation
Acute myeloid leukemia with maturation
Acute myelomonocytic leukemia
Acute monoblastic and monocytic leukemia
Acute erythroid leukemia
Acute megakaryoblastic leukemia
Acute basophilic leukemia
Acute panmyelosis with myelofibrosis
Myeloid sarcoma

Acute leukemia of ambiguous lineage
Undifferentiated acute leukemia
Bilineal acute leukemia
Biphenotypic acute leukemia

Table 8.3. Revised Realistic Pathologic Classification of acute myeloid leukemia.

Acute myeloid leukemia, *de novo*
Acute myeloid leukemia, not otherwise specified (NOS)
Acute myeloid leukemia with changes suggestive of
   t(8;21)(q22;q22)
Acute promyelocytic leukemia
Acute myeloid leukemia with abnormal eosinophils suggestive
   of inv(16)(p13q22) or t(16;16)(p13;q22)
Acute megakaryoblastic leukemia (childhood)
Acute myeloid leukemia with multilineage dysplasia
Acute myeloid leukemia, treatment-related

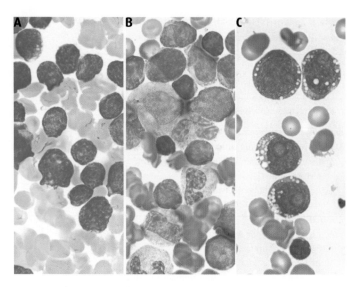

Figure 8.1. FAB types of acute lymphoblastic leukemia (ALL). (A) L1 morphology with uniform-sized blasts. (B) L2 ALL with more blast cell variation. (C) L3 blasts with more clumped nuclear chromatin, nucleoli, basophilic cytoplasm, and cytoplasmic vacuoles.

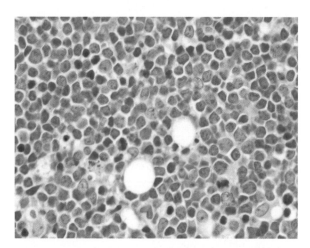

Figure 8.2. Bone marrow biopsy of precursor B-cell ALL with a monotonous population of small immature cells. The morphology of precursor T-cell ALL is similar and the immunophenotype of the blasts cannot be determined by the morphologic features alone.

Table 8.4. Common balanced cytogenetic translocations in acute leukemia.

	Cytogenetic abnormality	Genes
Precursor B-ALL		
	t(9;22)(q34;q11)	BCR/ABL
	11q23 translocations	MLL
	t(1;19)(q23;p13)	PBX/E2A
	t(12;21)(p13;q22)	TEL/AML1
Burkitt leukemia		
	t(8;14)(q24;q32)	MYC/IgH
	t(2;8)(p13;q24)	Igκ/MYC
	t(8;22)(q24;q11)	MYC/Igλ
T-ALL		
	t(10;14)(q24;q11)	HOX11/TCRδ
	t(7;10)(q35;q24)	TCRβ/HOX11
	t(1;14)(p33;q11)	TAL1/TCRα
	t(7;9)(q34;q32)	TCR/TAL2
	t(7;19)(q34;p13)	TCR/LYL1
	t(11;14)(p15;q11)	LMO1/TCRδ
	t(11;14)(p13;q11)	LMO2/TCRδ
	t(7;11)(q35;p13)	TCRβ/LMO2
	t(8;14)(q24;q11)	MYC/TCRδ
	t(1;7)(p34;q34)	LCK/TCR
	t(7;9)(q34;q34.3)	TCR/TAN1
	inv(14)(q11q32)	IgH or TCL1
AML		
	t(8;21)(q22;q22)	AML1/ETO
	t(3;21)(q26;q22)	EAP, MDS, or EVI1/AML1
	inv(16)(p13q22)/ t(16;16)(p13;q22)	CBFβ/MYH11
	t(15;17)(q22;q12)	PML/RARa
	t(11;17)(q13;q21)	NuMA/RARa
	t(11;17)(q23;q21)	PLZF/RARa
	t(5;17)(q35;q21)	NPM/RARa
	11q23 translocations	MLL
	t(6;9)(p23;q34)	DEK/CAN
	t(3;5)(q25;q34)	NPM/MLF1
	11p15 translocations	NUP98
	inv(3)(q21q26)	EVI1
	t(1;22)(p13;q13)	OTT/MAL

lymphomas. Other cases that would have been considered as ALL L3 in the past are now included in the Burkitt lymphoma/leukemia group (Table 8.2).

Precursor B-cell ALL is the most common type of ALL (Fig. 8.2). It characteristically expresses CD19, CD79a, cytoplasmic CD22 and TdT, and is usually CD10-positive (Khalidi *et al.*, 1999). Many of these markers can be effectively demonstrated in histologic material, if needed (Orazi *et al.*, 1994; Arber & Jenkins, 1996) (Fig. 8.3). The blast cells will also often express CD20 and CD34, but may be negative for these markers as well as CD45 and do not usually express surface immunoglobulin light or heavy chains.

Immunophenotypic subgroups of precursor B-cell ALL have separated cases based on expression of CD10 and cytoplasmic mu (Bene *et al.*, 1995), but these subgroups are not as significant as the detection of specific

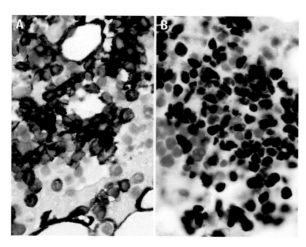

Figure 8.3. Immunohistochemistry of precursor B-cell ALL. (A) CD79a and (B) TdT nuclear positivity are detected.

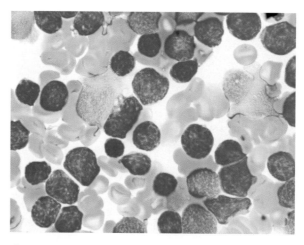

Figure 8.5. Precursor T-cell acute lymphoblastic leukemia. The blasts do not show distinctive morphologic features to suggest the T-cell immunophenotype.

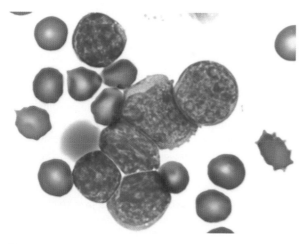

Figure 8.4. Pro-B (CD10-negative) ALL in an infant with t(4;11). The blasts showed aberrant expression of CD15, a common immunophenotype of this disease. They show more abundant cytoplasm than other types of ALL and may be mistaken for myeloblasts.

ALL-associated cytogenetic translocations (Wetzler *et al.*, 1999). Cytogenetic subgroups of precursor B-cell ALL include the t(9;22)(q34;q11), or the Philadelphia chromosome, which represents a fusion of the *BCR* and *ABL* genes. This abnormality occurs more commonly in adult ALL (20% adult versus <5% pediatric cases) and is frequently associated with aberrant expression of myeloid antigens, particularly CD13 and CD33, as well as expression of CD38 (Tabernero *et al.*, 2001). Abnormalities of the *MLL* gene on chromosome region 11q23, particularly t(4;11)(q21;q23), are associated with infant ALL and adult therapy-related ALL, a pro-B (CD10-negative) immunophenotype, and aberrant expression of CD15 and

CD65 (Ishizawa *et al.*, 2003) (Fig. 8.4). While the t(4;11) is associated with a poor prognosis, other *MLL* abnormalities, including 11q23 deletions that may not be easily detected on routine karyotype analysis, have varying prognostic significance (DiMartino & Cleary, 1999). The t(1;19)(q23;p13) and the t(12;21)(p13;q22) primarily occur in children, with the t(12;21) being extremely rare in adult ALL. The t(12;21) is not usually detectable by routine karyotype analysis, but lack of CD9 and CD20 expression, as well as other immunophenotypic abnormalities, have been reported to be associated with this abnormality (Borowitz *et al.*, 1998; De Zen *et al.*, 2000). Fluorescence *in situ* hybridization or polymerase chain reaction testing is needed to identify most cases of t(12;21) ALL (Borkhardt *et al.*, 1997), which are reported to represent at least 20% of childhood ALLs and are associated with a generally favorable prognosis.

Precursor T-cell ALL constitutes 15–20% of ALLs and is biologically similar, if not identical, to precursor T-cell lymphoblastic lymphoma (Gassmann *et al.*, 1997; Uckun *et al.*, 1998) (Fig. 8.5). Both are frequently associated with a mediastinal mass, and the presence of 25% or more blast cells in the bone marrow has been the traditional cutoff for considering a case as ALL rather than lymphoblastic lymphoma. The blast cell morphology of T-ALL is often identical to that of precursor B-cell ALL, although L2 blast features may be more common in T-ALL, and the immunophenotype of the leukemia cannot be predicted by morphologic features alone. The blast cells are usually positive for surface CD2, CD5, and CD7, as well as cytoplasmic CD3 and TdT, but may not express surface CD3 (Khalidi *et al.*, 1999). Some cases will demonstrate CD1a or dual expression of CD4 and CD8. Immunophenotypic subtypes of T-ALL have been proposed (Bene *et al.*, 1995), but are not usually considered

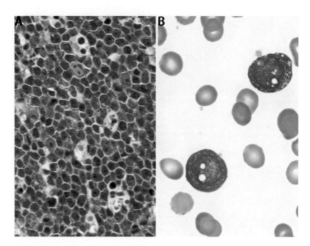

Figure 8.6. (A) Bone marrow biopsy showing complete replacement by Burkitt leukemia. The lymphocytes are fairly uniform in size, with nucleoli, a high mitotic rate, and numerous tingible-body macrophages imparting a "starry sky" appearance. (B) Precursor B-cell acute lymphoblastic leukemia with cytoplasmic vacuoles, mimicking Burkitt leukemia.

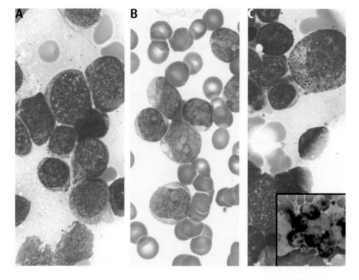

Figure 8.7. (A) Minimally differentiated acute myeloid leukemia (FAB M0). (B) Acute myeloid leukemia without maturation (FAB M1). (C) Acute myeloid leukemia with maturation (FAB M2). There are at least 10% of cells showing maturation. (*Inset*) The blasts are myeloperoxidase-positive by cytochemistry.

of significant prognostic value and are not included in the WHO classification. A variety of cytogenetic abnormalities, including translocations involving *TAL1* and the T-cell receptor genes, occur in T-ALL (Harrison, 2001). Some of these are summarized in Table 8.4.

Burkitt leukemia is a mature B-cell neoplasm that is the leukemic counterpart to Burkitt lymphoma (Dayton *et al.*,

1994). This type of leukemia overlaps with ALL-L3 of the FAB classification (Fig. 8.1), although cytoplasmic vacuoles of L3 are not required for the diagnosis of Burkitt leukemia. The blasts have more mature nuclear features than the other types of ALL, with clumped nuclear chromatin and multiple nucleoli. The blasts have darkly basophilic cytoplasm and often have prominent cytoplasmic vacuoles (Fig. 8.6). The vacuoles contain lipid and are oil red O-positive, although this special stain is not usually needed for diagnosis. In contrast to the other types of ALL, the leukemic cells of Burkitt leukemia are mature B cells and are TdT-negative. The cells express CD19, CD20, CD22, and surface light and heavy chains (Khalidi *et al.*, 1999). Cytoplasmic vacuoles may be seen in other types of ALL with more immature nuclear features and an immature lymphoid immunophenotype, but the designation of Burkitt leukemia should only be used for cases with a mature B-cell immunophenotype. The Burkitt cells are also CD10-positive and show a high proliferation rate (>90%) with Ki-67 staining. On biopsy material, the leukemic cells show a high mitotic rate with admixed tingible-body macrophages imparting a "starry sky" appearance (Fig. 8.6). Burkitt leukemia is associated with cytogenetic translocations involving the *C-MYC* gene on chromosome region 8q24, with t(8;14)(q24;q32), involving the immunoglobulin heavy chain gene, being the most common abnormality.

The classification of ALL does not separate the disease by age group, but there are significant clinical differences in the disease by age. The age groups can be generally divided into infant, childhood (and young adult), and adult ALL, with the childhood ALL having the best prognosis. ALL in young adults appears to behave in a manner that is similar to childhood disease. Infant ALL has a poor prognosis and is most commonly associated with abnormalities of the *MLL* gene, particularly t(4;11). Adult ALL has a higher association with the presence of t(9;22), which confers a poor prognosis. However, Philadelphia chromosome-negative ALL in adults also has a worse prognosis than similar disease in children, and patient age is an important prognostic factor in this disease that is not reflected by any of the classification systems.

Acute myeloid leukemia

The French–American–British Cooperative Group (FAB) classification of acute myeloid leukemia (AML) was originally a "pure" morphologic and cytochemical classification, but was later modified to include diseases that could only be recognized with additional ancillary techniques. Minimally differentiated acute myeloid leukemia (M0) (Fig. 8.7) is an acute leukemia with uniform blast cells without cytoplasmic granules or Auer rods and negative blast cell cytochemical reactions for myeloperoxidase, Sudan black B, and non-specific esterase (Bennett *et al.*, 1991; Cohen *et al.*, 1998). The myeloid lineage of the M0 blast cells is only recognizable by immunophenotyping methods, which usually show the blast cells to be CD13- and CD33-positive (Kotylo *et al.*, 2000). The blast cells should not express lymphoid specific antigens, but may be TdT-positive. A subset of cases will be myeloperoxidase-positive by immunophenotyping methods (Arber & Jenkins, 1996; Kotylo *et al.*, 2000). Without complete immunophenotyping studies, these cases may be misdiagnosed as acute lymphoblastic leukemia based on the negative cytochemical reactions.

Acute myeloid leukemias that are myeloperoxidase-positive and non-specific esterase-negative by cytochemistry are designated AML without maturation (M1) (Fig. 8.7), AML with maturation (M2) (Fig. 8.7), and acute promyelocytic leukemia (M3), with 10% or more bone marrow cells showing maturation to or beyond the promyelocyte level for a diagnosis of M2. Acute promyelocytic leukemia shows immature cells that are strongly myeloperoxidase-positive, but some cases may also show non-specific esterase positivity. There are two major morphologic categories of M3 leukemia, the hypergranular and hypogranular (microgranular) variants (Neame *et al.*, 1997) (Fig. 8.8). The hypergranular variant shows a proliferation of promyelocytes with granular cytoplasm and abundant Auer rods. These cells are more uniform in their level of differentiation than M2 leukemia, with relatively few cells with true blast cell morphology. The hypogranular variant may contain rare cells with many granules and Auer rods, but the majority of cells have very fine or indiscernible cytoplasmic granules without Auer rods, and folded, bilobate nuclei. Despite the apparent absence of cytoplasmic granules, this variant is also strongly myeloperoxidase-positive. The bilobate nuclei, abundant seemingly agranular cytoplasm, and possibility of non-specific esterase positivity may result in a misinterpretation of this variant as an acute myelomonocytic leukemia.

Acute myelomonocytic leukemia (M4) (Fig. 8.9) consists of a blast cell proliferation with folded nuclei, and some blast cells may have cytoplasmic granules and Auer rods. A subset of the blast cells are myeloperoxidase-positive, but the strong positivity of virtually all cells seen in M3 AML is not usually present. The blast cells are also non-specific esterase-positive, with 20–80% of bone marrow blast cells positive by definition. A subtype of M4 AML (acute myelomonocytic leukemia with eosinophilia, M4Eo) is included in the FAB classification that is associated with the presence of abnormal eosinophils with coarse basophilic granules (see Fig. 8.15).

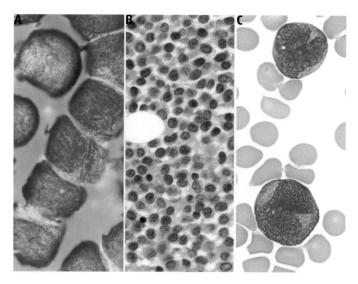

Figure 8.8. (A) Acute promyelocytic leukemia (FAB M3), hypergranular type with abundant Auer rods. (B) M3 biopsy. (C) M3, hypogranular type with folded nuclei, and small and indistinct granules.

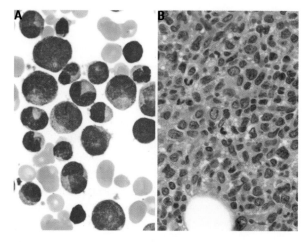

Figure 8.9. Acute myelomonocytic leukemia (FAB M4). A subset of the cells have monocytic features with folded nuclei on (A) the aspirate and (B) biopsy.

When over 80% of blast cells are positive for non-specific esterase, a diagnosis of acute monocytic leukemia (M5) is made. These cases may be myeloperoxidase-negative, but differ from M0 AML by their positivity for non-specific esterase. The blasts of M5 AML have abundant, often agranular cytoplasm, which may contain vacuoles. The blast nuclei may be round and uniform, or folded. Cases with more immature nuclear features in the bone marrow are termed M5a (Fig. 8.10), while those with evidence of monocytoid maturation in the bone marrow are termed M5b (Fig. 8.11). Monocyte maturation may be prominent in the

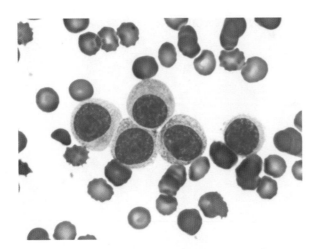

Figure 8.10. Acute monoblastic leukemia (FAB M5a), showing little evidence of maturation.

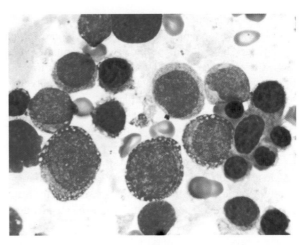

Figure 8.12. Acute erythroleukemia (FAB M6). There is a predominance of dysplastic erythroid precursors with admixed myeloblasts.

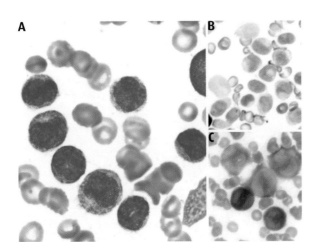

Figure 8.11. Acute monocytic leukemia (FAB M5b) with (A) evidence of maturation on the aspirate smear. (B) The blasts are cytochemically negative for myeloperoxidase, and (C) are virtually all positive for non-specific esterase.

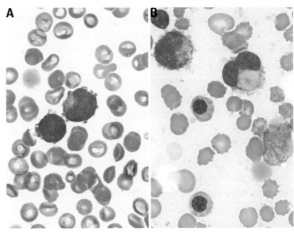

Figure 8.13. (A, B) Different examples of megakaryoblasts in acute megakaryoblastic leukemia (FAB M7).

peripheral blood in either type of M5 AML as well as in M4 AML, and the subclassification is best made on bone marrow specimens.

Erythroleukemia (M6) in the FAB classification is a myeloid blast cell proliferation that occurs in association with erythroid hyperplasia (Fig. 8.12). Erythroid precursors represent over 50% of the bone marrow cells, and blast cells are 30% or more of the non-erythroid elements for this diagnosis. Acute megakaryoblastic leukemia (M7) is a proliferation of blast cells that express megakaryocytic markers, such as CD41 or CD61, or are positive for platelet peroxidase by electron microscopy. The blast cells

are myeloperoxidase-negative, and may have a lymphoid appearance with friable cytoplasm with cytoplasmic blebs (Fig. 8.13). Marrow fibrosis is frequently present in this type of AML. Although morphologic features may suggest megakaryocytic differentiation, the diagnosis must be confirmed by immunophenotyping or electron microscopic studies.

The WHO and Realistic Pathologic Classifications of AML differ from the FAB classification in several areas. The blast cell count needed for a diagnosis of AML has been lowered to 20% in these systems, and some categories of disease do not have a minimum blast cell percentage. Also, the newer classifications include significant cytogenetic

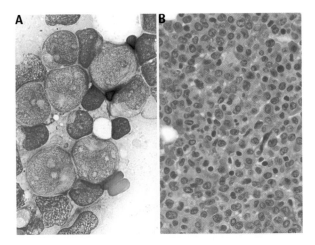

Figure 8.14. Acute myeloid leukemia with t(8;21). (A) The aspirate shows blasts with abundant cytoplasm and large pink granules. (B) An increase in normal-appearing eosinophils may be present, as seen on this biopsy.

disease groups, some of which are correlated with FAB groups, and there is less of an emphasis on cytochemical studies for many of the newer disease categories. Both systems recognize categories of AML with recurring cytogenetic abnormalities.

Acute myeloid leukemias with recurrent genetic abnormalities

Several recurring cytogenetic abnormalities occur in AML, and characteristic morphologic, cytochemical, and/or immunophenotypic features may suggest some of these abnormalities (Arber *et al.*, 2003b). These leukemias may occur at any age, but represent a higher percentage of AMLs in children. AML with t(8;21)(q22;q22) is associated with a fusion of the *AML1* (or *CBFα*) gene on chromosome 21 and the *ETO* (or *MTG8*) gene on chromosome 8 (Nisson *et al.*, 1992). This type of AML represents a subset of M2 AMLs in the FAB classification and represents 5–10% of all AMLs and up to one-third of AMLs with M2 features. Extramedullary myeloid tumors (also known as myeloid or granulocytic sarcomas or chloromas) are more common with this type of AML. The bone marrow and peripheral blood blast cells show promyelocytic maturation with large azurophilic granules, and large salmon-colored granules are identifiable in some cells (Nakamura *et al.*, 1997) (Fig. 8.14). Auer rods are frequently present and an associated increase in normal-appearing eosinophils is common. Maturing granulocytes may show abnormalities of nuclear lobation, but dysplastic changes of other cell lines are not usually present, unless the leukemia is

therapy-related (Arber *et al.*, 2002). The blast cells are myeloperoxidase- and Sudan black B-positive, and are usually non-specific esterase-negative. The blasts usually express myeloid-associated antigens (Khalidi *et al.*, 1998), such as CD13 and CD33, but myeloid antigen-negative cases that are myeloperoxidase-positive have been rarely reported (Arber *et al.*, 1997). The blasts are characteristically CD34-positive and approximately two-thirds of cases aberrantly express the B-cell-associated markers CD19 and PAX5 without other lymphoid antigen expression (Kita *et al.*, 1992). A subset of cases will also express CD56, and such expression has been associated with a worse prognosis (Baer *et al.*, 1997). The blast cells may be below 20% in some cases, but with the characteristic morphologic and immunophenotypic features and the presence of t(8;21) these cases should be considered acute leukemias rather than myelodysplastic syndromes. This type of AML has an intermediate to favorable prognosis with current therapy.

AML with inv(16)(p13q22) or t(16;16)(p13;q22) is associated with a fusion of the *CBFβ* and *MYH11* genes on chromosome 16 (Le Beau *et al.*, 1983). This leukemia generally corresponds to AML-M4Eo in the FAB classification, although some cases are non-specific esterase-negative and may be termed M2 in that system. This leukemia represents approximately 10% of AMLs, and is biologically related to the t(8;21) AMLs, with both resulting in an abnormality of the core-binding factor complex that is required for normal hematopoiesis. The blast cells usually show myelomonocytic features with folded nuclei, with or without cytoplasmic granules and Auer rods. A subset of blasts is usually myeloperoxidase- and Sudan black B-positive and non-specific esterase-positive, but the cytochemical profile is less important than the identification of abnormal eosinophils in these cases. The majority of cases of AML with inv(16) will show an increase in eosinophils that contain abnormal coarse basophilic granules (Fig. 8.15). The presence of an increase in normal-appearing eosinophils is not sufficient to make this diagnosis. These eosinophils are chloroacetate esterase-positive, in contrast to the negative cytochemical reaction in normal eosinophils, but cytochemical studies are not usually necessary for this diagnosis. Abnormal eosinophils may not be present in a significant minority of cases (Arber *et al.*, 2003b), and they are less frequent in peripheral blood samples than in the bone marrow. The blast cells express myelomonocytic antigens, and a subset aberrantly co-express the T-cell-associated antigen CD2. Similar to t(8;21) AML, bone marrow blast cells may be below 20% in some cases, but with the characteristic morphologic features and the presence of inv(16) or t(16;16), these cases should be considered

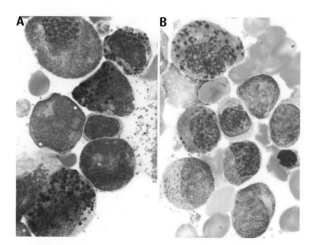

Figure 8.15. (A, B) Acute myeloid leukemia with inv(16) or t(16;16). Blasts with monocytic features are present with eosinophils and eosinophil precursors. Many of the eosinophils have abnormal, large basophilic granules that are characteristic of this cytogenetic abnormality.

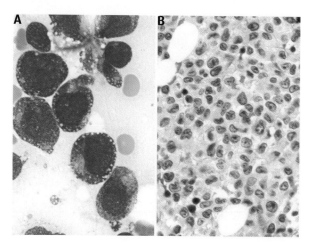

Figure 8.16. Acute myeloid leukemia with 11q23 abnormalities. This case shows prominent monocytic features on (A) the aspirate and (B) biopsy.

acute leukemias rather than myelodysplastic syndromes. This type of AML has a favorable prognosis.

Acute promyelocytic leukemia, or AML with t(15;17)(q22;q12) and variants, is associated with an abnormality of the *RARα* gene of chromosome 17, which is fused to the *PML* gene of chromosome 15 in the vast majority of cases (Melnick & Licht, 1999), This leukemia corresponds to AML-M3 of the FAB classification and represents 5–10% of all AMLs. A high percentage of patients with this type of AML will present with disseminated intravascular coagulopathy (DIC). The morphologic features of this disease are described above for FAB M3 AML (Fig. 8.8). The blasts are characteristically positive for the myeloid-associated antigens CD13 and CD33, but are usually negative for HLA-DR and CD34. Some cases may show a subset of HLA-DR-positive cells, but the general decrease in HLA-DR expression by the blast cells of acute promyelocytic leukemia differs from most other AMLs (Guglielmi *et al.*, 1998). The blast cells also frequently aberrantly co-express CD2 and/or CD9. Variant *RARα* translocation partners include *PLZF* at 11q23, *NuMA* at 11q13, and *NPM* at 5q35. More recently, a *STAT 5b/RARα* fusion resulting from an interstitial deletion of chromosome 17 has also been described. Cases that lack an *RARα* translocation, or that have a translocation involving *PLZF* or *STAT 5b*, do not respond to all-*trans*-retinoic acid and require a different therapeutic approach.

These variants have features that are generally similar to t(15;17) AML, but some morphologic differences occur with t(11;17)(q23;q21) (Sainty *et al.*, 2000). This subtype shows

abnormalities of maturing neutrophils with clumped, condensed nuclear chromatin and monolobate or bilobate "Pelger-like" cells. Similar to other types of AML with recurring cytogenetic abnormalities, bone marrow blast cells may be below 20% in some cases, but with the characteristic morphologic features and the presence of an *RARα*-associated translocation, these cases should be considered acute leukemias rather than myelodysplastic syndromes. This type of AML has a favorable prognosis when treated with therapeutic regimens that include all-*trans*-retinoic acid (Tallman *et al.*, 1997), with the exception of cases with the cytogenetic abnormalities mentioned above.

The WHO classification also recognizes a category of AML with 11q23 abnormalities that are associated with translocations and other abnormalities involving the *MLL* gene of chromosome 11. Abnormalities of *MLL* represent approximately 5% of all AMLs and include subgroups of infant AML, *de novo* AML in other age groups, and therapy-related AML, particularly following treatment with DNA topoisomerase II inhibitors. The blast cells usually show monocytic features (Fig. 8.16), with varying degrees of nonspecific esterase positivity by cytochemistry, and would be considered M4 or M5 AMLs in the FAB classification. The blasts express various myelomonocytic-associated antigens (Baer *et al.*, 1998). A variety of translocation partners are described for the *MLL* gene, as well as other abnormalities not associated with translocations, including partial tandem duplication of the gene. The prognosis for this leukemia type is intermediate to poor, and varies by the type of *MLL* abnormality and clinical situation. The t(9;11)(p22;q23) in AML appears to indicate an improved

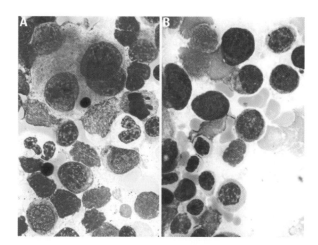

Figure 8.17. (A, B) Acute myeloid leukemia with multilineage dysplasia. Blast cells are admixed with dysplastic neutrophils, erythroid precursors, and megakaryocytes.

outcome when compared to other *MLL* translocations (Mrozek *et al.*, 1997). Because of the lack of specific morphologic, cytochemical, or immunophenotypic features for this leukemia type, and the prognostic differences within this group, this is not a specific leukemia type in the Realistic Pathologic Classification, but identification of an *MLL* abnormality should be recognized as a prognostically significant feature of AML. Therapy-related cases should be designated as such and should be separated from *de novo* AMLs with *MLL* abnormalities.

Acute myeloid leukemia with multilineage dysplasia and therapy-related acute myeloid leukemia

AML with multilineage dysplasia and therapy-related AML are diseases that usually show dysplastic changes in the non-blast marrow and peripheral blood elements. The WHO classification defines AML with multilineage dysplasia as 20% or more bone marrow or peripheral blood blast cells with 50% or more dysplastic cells in at least two cell lines (erythroid, granulocytic, or megakaryocytic) (Fig. 8.17). The 50% cutoff for dysplastic changes is arbitrary and excludes some cases with definite associated dysplastic changes. Dysplastic changes may be seen in both peripheral blood and bone marrow samples. Red cell changes include anisopoikilocytosis of peripheral blood red cells, including hypochromic teardrop-shaped cells and macrocytes, dimorphic red cell populations of the blood, nuclear-cytoplasmic asynchrony of red cell precursors, megaloblastic changes, and irregularities of red cell precursor nuclei. Megaloblastic changes differ from a "left shift" of erythroid

cells by the presence of more immature nuclear chromatin, often associated with more mature, red-staining erythroid cell cytoplasm. Nuclear irregularities, including multinucleation, nuclear blebs, and irregular nuclear contours, are commonly seen in dysplastic erythroid precursors. Granulocyte dysplasia is most easily recognized in the more mature granulocyte forms of the blood and marrow. These changes include uneven cytoplasmic granulation or completely agranular mature neutrophils. Nuclear changes include clumping of nuclear chromatin that is usually associated with abnormalities of nuclear lobation, particularly monolobate or bilobate nuclei ("pseudo-Pelger–Huët" cells). Peripheral blood platelets may show variation in platelet size with hypogranular platelets. Megakaryocytes may show great variation in size with detached, hyperlobulated nuclei or hypolobated or monolobated forms with hyperchromatic nuclei. Multilineage dysplasia-associated AML does not show specific blast cell morphologic features, and can include all types of FAB AMLs, although FAB-M3 leukemia with multilineage dysplasia is unusual. Therefore, there are no specific cytochemical or immunophenotypic features of the blast cells for this disease category.

AML with multilineage dysplasia may occur *de novo* or may follow known myelodysplasia (Gahn *et al.*, 1996). Both types show an increased frequency of complex cytogenetic abnormalities, deletions on chromosomes 5 or 7, trisomies, or abnormalities of chromosome band 3q21. AML with multilineage dysplasia is generally associated with a poor prognosis, and separation of *de novo* cases and those arising from myelodysplasia does not appear to have clinical relevance (Arber *et al.*, 2003a).

Therapy-related AML is further subdivided in the WHO classification into alkylating agent-related and topoisomerase II inhibitor-related types. Alkylating agent-related disease (Fig. 8.18) usually occurs 5–7 years after therapy, and shows morphologic and cytogenetic changes similar to AML with multilineage dysplasia, with deletions of chromosome 5 and 7 common (Pedersen-Bjergaard *et al.*, 2000). Topoisomerase II inhibitor-related disease (Fig. 8.18) generally has a shorter latency period of 2–3 years, tends to have monocytic features, and may or may not have associated multilineage dysplasia. Abnormalities of the *MLL* gene of 11q23 and the *AML1* gene of 21q22 are commonly present in these cases, but a variety of other abnormalities, including inv(16) and t(15;17), may also be seen (Rowley & Olney, 2002). Therapy-related acute lymphoblastic leukemia with *MLL* abnormalities may also occur, but is not included in any of the current acute leukemia classification systems (Ishizawa *et al.*, 2003). Therapy-related AML is generally associated with a poor prognosis. Many patients receive a combination of therapies that may include both alkylating

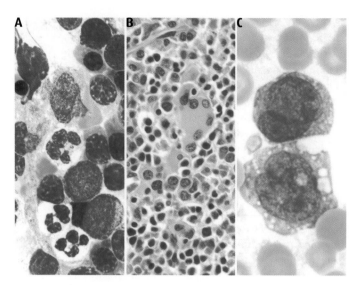

Figure 8.18. Therapy-related acute myeloid leukemia following alkylating agent therapy: (A) aspirate; (B), biopsy. This leukemia shows features that are similar to acute myeloid leukemia with multilineage dysplasia. (C) Therapy-related acute myeloid leukemia following topoisomerase II inhibitors. This leukemia shows prominent monocytic features and has an 11q23 abnormality.

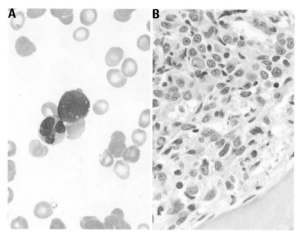

Figure 8.19. Acute megakaryoblastic leukemia of infancy with t(1;22). The blasts have similar features to other megakaryoblasts on the aspirate (A) and the biopsy (B) is fibrotic, similar to the other forms of this disease.

and topoisomerase II inhibitors, or develop therapy-related AML following radiation or administration of other drug types, and it is often difficult to obtain the specifics of the prior therapy at the time of diagnosis. For this reason, the Realistic Pathologic Classification does not subdivide therapy-related AMLs.

Acute myeloid leukemia not otherwise categorized

Despite its name, AML not otherwise categorized in the WHO classification contains ten different categories, listed in Table 8.2. These categories largely follow the original FAB categories for disease, but they do not include cases with any of the recurrent genetic abnormalities or with multilineage dysplasia. There is little if any clinical significance to these designations (Arber *et al.*, 2003a), and these cases are largely included in the category of AML not otherwise specified (NOS) in the Realistic Pathologic Classification.

One disease that is separated from AML not otherwise categorized in the Realistic Pathologic Classification is acute megakaryoblastic leukemia. Acute megakaryoblastic leukemia of the FAB classification (M7) appears to represent two clinical diseases, one in young children and one in adults (Ribeiro *et al.*, 1993; Gassmann & Löffler, 1995). The adult disease is associated with organomegaly

and multilineage dysplasia, and should be classified as AML with multilineage dysplasia (Fig. 8.13). An association with mediastinal non-seminomatous germ cell tumors has been reported with adult acute megakaryoblastic leukemia (Orazi *et al.*, 1993). *De novo* acute megakaryoblastic leukemia is an uncommon disease representing 1% or less of AMLs. It may be associated with Down syndrome, often following resolution of a transient myeloproliferative disorder occurring at around 2 years of age, or may be associated with t(1;22)(p13;q13), which usually occurs as a sole abnormality in the first six months of life (Lion *et al.*, 1992; Lu *et al.*, 1993) (Fig. 8.19). Both diseases show a blast cell proliferation with uniform, often "lymphoid" cells with varying amounts of basophilic cytoplasm without Auer rods. Cytoplasmic blebs may be present, but are not specific enough for use as an absolute diagnostic criterion. The blast cells are myeloperoxidase- and Sudan black B-negative, but may be positive for the non-specific esterase alpha-naphthyl acetate esterase (sodium-fluoride sensitive). The blasts may express myeloid-associated antigens, but should also express at least two megakaryocyte-associated antigens, such as CD41, CD42, CD61, von Willebrand factor, or *Ulex europaeus*. The detection of platelet peroxidase by electron microscopy is also sufficient for assignment of megakaryocyte lineage in these cases. The prognosis for acute megakaryoblastic leukemia is poor.

Acute panmyelosis with myelofibrosis (APMF) (Fig. 8.20) is considered by some authors to be an exceedingly rare subtype of acute myeloid leukemia and corresponds to less than 1% of cases. The WHO criteria for the diagnosis of APMF include panmyelosis, significant marrow

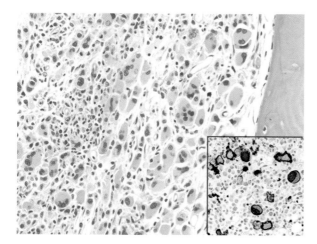

Figure 8.20. Acute panmyelosis with myelofibrosis. The biopsy shows features similar to acute megakaryoblastic leukemia, but with fewer blast cells. (*Inset*) CD42b stain, highlighting numerous abnormal megakaryocytes.

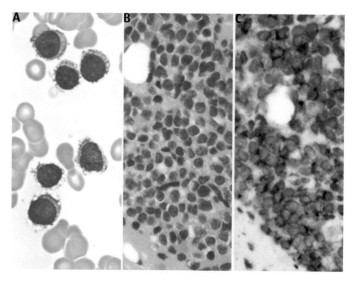

Figure 8.21. Pure erythroid leukemia: (A) aspirate; (B) biospy. The leukemia cells are all of erythroid lineage and show glycophorin expression by immunohistochemistry (C).

fibrosis, pancytopenia, normal erythrocyte morphology, lack of splenomegaly, and a rapidly fatal course. Bone marrow aspiration is usually unsuccessful and the bone marrow biopsy supplemented with immunohistology is required for appropriate characterization.

Most cases of APMF are characterized by a hypercellular, diffusely fibrotic bone marrow with an increased number of multilineage immature hematopoietic elements, and conspicuously dysplastic megakaryocytes predominantly of small size showing variable degrees of atypia including the presence of hypolobated or nonlobated nuclei with dispersed chromatin. Foci of blasts are found scattered throughout the marrow. The overall frequency of blasts in APMF marrows is uncertain. In a recent study based on bone marrow biopsy, we found a blast frequency comprised between 10% and 25% with a median value of 22.5% (Orazi *et al.*, 2005); however, its precise determination is not considered a diagnostic requirement, according to the WHO system. Most of the blasts express CD34 and are negative for the megakaryocyte-associated markers (Orazi *et al.*, 2005). The course is rapidly fatal, often terminating with an overtly leukemic myeloid phase, or rarely with a lymphoblastic malignancy. In the terminal stage, splenomegaly may be observed, which usually results from leukemic infiltration of the red pulp. The disease usually occurs in adults, but rare cases have been described in children. The main differential diagnosis is with myelodysplastic syndrome with fibrosis associated with an excess of blasts, cases of AML with multilineage dysplasia with a low blast frequency (see also Chapter 7), and acute megakaryoblastic leukemia with a "dry tap." Distinction, in some of these cases, may be

arbitrary and clinically irrelevant, and thus some authors do not consider this to be a distinct entity.

The category of acute erythroid leukemia in the WHO classification has been expanded from the original FAB M6 category. One type of erythroid leukemia has a definition similar to that of the FAB category, with over 50% erythroid cells and an increase in myeloblasts to 20% or more of non-erythroid cells (Fig. 8.12). The second type represents a true proliferation of erythroid cells without a required increase in myeloblasts (Fig. 8.21). These cases are considered erythroid leukemia if erythroblasts represent over 80% of marrow cells. These erythroblasts often have vacuolated, basophilic cytoplasm and the vacuoles are PAS-positive. The vast majority of cases of either type of erythroid leukemia are associated with multilineage dysplasia and are designated as a type of myelodysplasia or AML with multilineage dysplasia in the Realistic Pathologic Classification.

Biphenotypic acute leukemia

Many acute leukemias aberrantly express antigens that are unexpected for the leukemia type (Fig. 8.22). As described previously, some of these aberrant antigen profiles are useful in the diagnosis of specific disease types, and the presence of aberrant antigen expression does not usually equate to biphenotypic or mixed-lineage acute leukemia.

Table 8.5. Modified EGIL scoring system for biphenotypic acute leukemia. A diagnosis of biphenotypic acute leukemia requires a score of over 2 points for the myeloid and one of the lymphoid lineages.

Points	B lineage	T lineage	Myeloid lineage
2	CD79a	CD3 (m/cyt)	anti-MPO (monoclonal)
	cyt IgM	anti-TCR α/β	MPO cytochemistry
	cyt CD22	anti-TCR γ/δ	
1	CD19	CD2	CD117
	CD10	CD5	CD13
	CD20	CD8	CD33
		CD10	CD65s
			anti-MPO (polyclonal)
0.5	TdT	TdT	CD14
	CD24	CD7	CD15
		CD1a	CD64

m, membrane; cyt, cytoplasmic

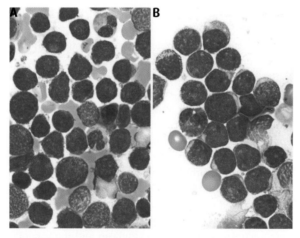

Figure 8.22. Biphenotypic acute leukemia. (A) Precursor B/myeloid lineage; (B) precursor T/myeloid lineage. Both show variable blasts, some with granules and some with a more lymphoid appearance. This diagnosis is made based on the immunophenotypic criteria described in the text.

The European Group for the Immunological Classification of Leukaemias (EGIL) has proposed criteria for lineage assignment in acute leukemia and a modified version of those criteria is shown in Table 8.5 (Bene *et al.*, 1995; European Group for the Immunological Classification of Leukaemias, 1998; Arber *et al.*, 2001). This system requires more than two points for each lineage (myeloid and one lymphoid) for a diagnosis of biphenotypic acute leukemia. Using this system, less than 5% of acute leukemias would

be considered biphenotypic. The WHO classification further divides cases into bilineal acute leukemia, where two morphologically distinct blast cell populations are identified, and biphenotypic acute leukemia, if distinct populations are not identified. In our experience, even cases with a bilineal morphologic pattern show at least one of the cell populations to express dual antigens. The significance of biphenotypic antigen expression is unclear. A significant percentage of cases will express precursor B-cell antigens and myeloid-associated antigens and demonstrate t(9;22). Such cases may be better designated Philadelphia chromosome-positive acute lymphoblastic leukemia with aberrant myeloid antigen expression, since this is an already well-recognized disease type (Tabernero *et al.*, 2001). The t(4;11) is also common in this group, and these cases are also similar to ALLs with this cytogenetic abnormality. Although the prognosis is generally poor for cases of biphenotypic acute leukemia, this prognosis may be more related to the associated cytogenetic abnormalities than to the immunophenotype.

Acute undifferentiated leukemia

Despite extensive immunophenotyping, a very small percentage of acute leukemias will not express sufficient lineage-specific markers for classification as myeloid or lymphoid lineage. These leukemias may show quite variable blast cell morphology, and may express non-specific antigens such as CD34, TdT, and CD7. By cytochemistry, the cells are negative for myeloperoxidase, Sudan black B, and non-specific esterase. They are generally considered to have a poor prognosis.

REFERENCES

Arber, D. A. (2001). Realistic pathologic classification of acute myeloid leukemias. *American Journal of Clinical Pathology*, **115**, 552–60.

Arber, D. A. & Jenkins, K. A. (1996). Paraffin section immunophenotype of acute leukemias in bone marrow specimens. *American Journal of Clinical Pathology*, **106**, 462–8.

Arber, D. A., Glackin, C., Lowe, G., Medeiros, L. J., & Slovak, M. L. (1997). Presence of t(8;21)(q22;q22) in myeloperoxidase-positive, myeloid surface antigen-negative acute myeloid leukemia. *American Journal of Clinical Pathology*, **107**, 68–73.

Arber, D. A., Snyder, D. S., Fine, M., Dagis, A., Niland, J., & Slovak, M. L. (2001). Myeloperoxidase immunoreactivity in adult acute lymphoblastic leukemia. *American Journal of Clinical Pathology*, **116**, 25–33.

Arber, D. A., Slovak, M. L., Popplewell, L., Bedell, V., Ikle, D., & Rowley, J. D. (2002). Therapy-related acute myeloid leukemia/myelodysplasia with balanced 21q22 translocations. *American Journal of Clinical Pathology*, **117**, 306–13.

Arber, D. A., Carter, N. H., Ikle, D., & Slovak, M. L. (2003a). Value of combined morphologic, cytochemical, and immunophenotypic features in predicting recurrent cytogenetic abnormalities in acute myeloid leukemia. *Human Pathology*, **34**, 479–83.

Arber, D. A., Stein, A. S., Carter, N. H., Ikle D., Forman, S. J., & Slovak, M. L. (2003b). Prognostic impact of acute myeloid leukemia classification: importance of detection of recurring cytogenetic abnormalities and multilineage dysplasia on survival. *American Journal of Clinical Pathology*, **119**, 672–80.

Baer, M. R., Stewart, C. C., Lawrence, D., *et al.* (1997). Expression of the neural cell adhesion molecule CD56 is associated with short remission duration and survival in acute myeloid leukemia with t(8;21)(q22;q22). *Blood*, **90**, 1643–8.

Baer, M. R., Stewart, C. C., Lawrence, D., *et al.* (1998). Acute myeloid leukemia with 11q23 translocations: myelomonocytic immunophenotype by multiparameter flow cytometry. *Leukemia*, **12**, 317–25.

Bene, M. C., Castoldi, G., Knapp, W., *et al.* (1995). Proposal for the immunologic classification of acute leukemias. *Leukemia*, **9**, 1783–6.

Bennett, J. M., Catovsky, D., Daniel, M. T., *et al.* (1976). Proposals for the classification of the acute leukemias. *British Journal of Haematology*, **33**, 451–8.

Bennett, J. M., Catovsky, D., Daniel, M. T., *et al.* (1981). The morphologic classification of acute lymphoblastic leukaemia: concordance among observers and clinical correlations. *British Journal of Haematology*, **47**, 553–61.

Bennett, J. M., Catovsky, D., Daniel, M. T., *et al.* (1985a). Proposed revised criteria for the classification of acute myeloid leukemia: a report of the French–American–British Cooperative Group. *Annals of Internal Medicine*, **103**, 620–5.

Bennett, J. M., Catovsky, D., Daniel, M. T., *et al.* (1985b). Criteria for the diagnosis of acute leukemia of megakaryocytic lineage (M7): a report of the French–American–British Cooperative Group. *Annals of Internal Medicine*, **103**, 460–2.

Bennett, J. M., Catovsky, D., Daniel, M. T., *et al.* (1991). Proposal for the recognition of minimally differentiated acute myeloid leukaemia (AML-M0). *British Journal of Haematology*, **78**, 325–9.

Borkhardt, A., Cazzaniga, G., Viehmann, S., *et al.* (1997). Incidence and clinical relevance of TEL/AML1 fusion genes in children with acute lymphoblastic leukemia enrolled in the German and Italian multicenter therapy trials. Associazione Italiana Ematologia Oncologia Pediatrica and the Berlin–Frankfurt–Munster Study Group. *Blood*, **90**, 571–7.

Borowitz, M. J., Rubnitz, J., Nash, M., Pullen, D. J., & Camitta B. (1998). Surface antigen phenotype can predict TEL-AML1 rearrangement in childhood B-precursor ALL: a Pediatric Oncology Group study. *Leukemia*, **12**, 1764–70.

Cohen, P. L., Hoyer, J. D., Kurtin, P. J., Dewald, G. W., & Hanson, C. A. (1998). Acute myeloid leukemia with minimal differentiation: a multiparameter study. *American Journal of Clinical Pathology*, **109**, 32–8.

Dayton, V. D., Arthur, D. C., Gajl-Peczalska, K. J., & Brunning, R. (1994). L3 acute lymphoblastic leukemia: comparison with small noncleaved cell lymphoma involving the bone marrow. *American Journal of Clinical Pathology*, **101**, 130–9.

De Zen, L., Orfao, A., Cazzaniga, G., *et al.* (2000). Quantitative multiparametric immunophenotyping in acute lymphoblastic leukemia: correlation with specific genotype. I. ETV6/AML1 ALLs identification. *Leukemia*, **14**, 1225–31.

DiMartino, J. F. & Cleary, M. L. (1999). MLL rearrangements in hematological malignancies: lessons from clinical and biological studies. *British Journal of Haematology*, **106**, 614–24.

European Group for the Immunological Classification of Leukaemias. (1998). The value of c-kit in the diagnosis of biphenotypic acute leukemia. *Leukemia*. **12**, 2038.

Gahn B., Haase, D., Unterhalt, M., Drescher, M., *et al.* (1996). *De novo* AML with dysplastic hematopoiesis: cytogenetic and prognostic significance. *Leukemia*, **10**, 946–51.

Gassmann, W. & Löffler, H. (1995). Acute megakaryoblastic leukaemia. *Leukemia and Lymphoma*, **18**, 69–73.

Gassmann, W., Löffler, H., Thiel, E., *et al.* (1997). Morphological and cytochemical findings in 150 cases of T-lineage acute lymphoblastic leukaemia in adults. *British Journal of Haematology*, **97**, 372–82.

Guglielmi, C., Martelli, M. P., Diverio, D., *et al.* (1998). Immunophenotype of adult and childhood acute promyelocytic leukaemia: correlation with morphology, type of PML gene breakpoint and clinical outcome. A cooperative Italian study on 196 cases. *British Journal of Haematology*, **102**, 1035–41.

Harris, N. L., Jaffe, E. S., Diebold, J., *et al.* (1999). The World Health Organization Classification of neoplastic diseases of the hematopoietic and lymphoid tissues: report of the Clinical Advisory Committee meeting, Airlie House, Virginia, November 1997. *Journal of Clinical Oncology*, **17**, 3835–49.

Harrison, C. J. (2001). Acute lymphoblastic leukaemia. *Best Practice & Research: Clinical Haematology*, **14**, 593–607.

Ishizawa, S., Slovak, M. L., Popplewell, L., *et al.* (2003). High frequency of pro-B acute lymphoblastic leukemia in adults with secondary leukemia with 11q23 abnormalities. *Leukemia*, **17**, 1091–5.

Jaffe, E. S., Harris, N. L., Stein, H., & Vardiman, J. W., eds. (2001). *World Health Organization Classification of Tumours: Pathology and Genetics of Tumours of Haematopoietic and Lymphoid Tissues.* Lyon: IARC Press.

Khalidi, H. S., Medeiros, L. J., Chang, K. L., Brynes, R. K., Slovak, M. L., & Arber, D. A. (1998). The immunophenotype of adult acute myeloid leukemia: high frequency of lymphoid antigen expression and comparison of immunophenotype, French–American–British classification, and karyotypic abnormalities. *American Journal of Clinical Pathology*, **109**, 211–20.

Khalidi, H. S., Chang, K. L., Medeiros, L. J., *et al.* (1999). Acute lymphoblastic leukemia: survey of immunophenotype, French–American–British classification, frequency of myeloid antigen expression, and karyotypic abnormalities in 210 pediatric and adult cases. *American Journal of Clinical Pathology*, **111**, 467–76.

Kita, K., Nakase, K., Miwa, H., *et al.* (1992). Phenotypical characteristics of acute myelocytic leukemia associated with the t(8;21)(q22;q22) chromosomal abnormality: frequent expression of immature B-cell antigen CD19 together with stem cell antigen CD34. *Blood*, **80**, 470–7.

Kotylo, P. K., Seo, I. S., Smith, F. O., *et al.* (2000). Flow cytometric immunophenotypic characterization of pediatric and adult minimally differentiated acute myeloid leukemia (AML-M0). *American Journal of Clinical Pathology*, **113**, 193–200.

Le Beau, M. M., Larson, R. A., Bitter, M. A., Vardiman, J. W., Golomb, H. M., & Rowley, J. D. (1983). Association of an inversion of chromosome 16 and abnormal marrow eosinophils in acute myelomonocytic leukemia. *New England Journal of Medicine*, **309**, 630–6.

Lion, T., Haas, O. A., Harbott, J., *et al.* (1992). The translocation t(1;22)(p13;q13) is a nonrandom marker specifically associated with acute megakaryocytic leukemia in young children. *Blood*, **79**, 3325–30.

Lu, G., Altman, A. J., & Benn, P. A. (1993). Review of the cytogenetic changes in acute megakaryoblastic leukemia: one disease or several? *Cancer Genetics and Cytogenetics*, **67**, 81–9.

Manaloor, E. J., Neiman, R. S., Heilman, D. K., *et al.* (2000). Immunohistochemistry can be used to subtype acute myeloid leukemia in routinely processed bone marrow biopsy specimens: Comparison with flow cytometry. *American Journal of Clinical Pathology*, **113**, 814–22.

Melnick, A. & Licht, J. D. (1999). Deconstructing a disease: RARa, its fusion partners, and their roles in the pathogenesis of acute promyelocytic leukemia. *Blood*, **93**, 3167–215.

Mrozek, K., Heinonen, K., Lawrence, D., *et al.* (1997). Adult patients with *de novo* acute myeloid leukemia and t(9;11)(p22;q23) have a superior outcome to patients with other translocations involving band 11q23: a Cancer and Leukemia Group B study. *Blood*, **90**, 4532–8.

Nakamura, H., Kuriyama, K., Sadamori, N., *et al.* (1997). Morphological subtyping of acute myeloid leukemia with maturation (AML-M2): homogeneous pink-colored cytoplasm of mature neutrophils is most characteristic of AML-M2 with t(8;21). *Leukemia*, **11**, 651–5.

Neame, P. B., Soamboonsrup, P., Leber, B., *et al.* (1997). Morphology of acute promyelocytic leukemia with cytogenetic or molecular evidence for the diagnosis: characterization of additional microgranular variants. *American Journal of Hematology*, **6**, 131–42.

Nisson, P. E., Watkins, P. C., & Sacchi, N. (1992). Transcriptionally active chimeric gene derived from the fusion of the AML1 gene and a novel gene on chromosome 8 in t(8;21) leukemic cells. *Cancer Genetics and Cytogenetics*, **63**, 81–8.

Orazi, A., Neiman, R. S., Ulbright, T. M., Heerema, N. A., John, K., & Nichols, C. R. (1993). Hematopoietic precursor cells within the yolk sac tumor component are the source of secondary hematopoietic malignancies in patients with mediastinal germ cell tumors. *Cancer*, **71**, 3873–81.

Orazi, A., Cotton, J., Cattoretti, G., *et al.* (1994). Terminal deoxynucleotidyl transferase staining in acute leukemia and normal bone marrow in routinely processed paraffin sections. *American Journal of Clinical Pathology*, **102**, 640–5.

Orazi, A., O'Malley, D. P., Jiang, J., *et al.* (2005). Acute panmyelosis with myelofibrosis: an entity distinct from acute megakaryoblastic leukemia. *Modern Pathology*, **18**, 603–14.

Pedersen-Bjergaard, J., Andersen, M. K., & Christiansen, D. H. (2000). Therapy-related acute myeloid leukemia and myelodysplasia after high-dose chemotherapy and autologous stem cell transplantation. *Blood*, **95**, 3273–9.

Ribeiro, R. C., Oliveira, M. S., Fairclough, D., *et al.* (1993). Acute megakaryoblastic leukemia in children and adolescents: a retrospective analysis of 24 cases. *Leukemia and Lymphoma*, **10**, 299–306.

Rowley, J. D. & Olney, H. J. (2002). International workshop on the relationship of prior therapy to balanced chromosome aberrations in therapy-related myelodysplastic syndromes and acute leukemia: overview report. *Genes, Chromosomes and Cancer*, **33**, 331–45.

Sainty, D., Liso, V., Cantu-Rajnoldi, A., *et al.* (2000). A new morphologic classification system for acute promyelocytic leukemia distinguishes cases with underlying *PLZF/RARA* gene rearrangements. *Blood*, **96**, 1287–96.

Tabernero, M. D., Bortoluci, A. M., Alaejos, I., *et al.* (2001). Adult precursor B-ALL with BCR/ABL gene rearrangements displays a unique immunophenotype based on the pattern of CD10, CD34, CD13 and CD38 expression. *Leukemia*, **15**, 406–14.

Tallman, M. S., Andersen, J. W., Schiffer, C. A., *et al.* (1997). All-*trans*-retinoic acid in acute promyelocytic leukemia. *New England Journal of Medicine*, **337**, 1021–8.

Uckun, F. M., Sensel, M. G., Sun, L., *et al.* (1998). Biology and treatment of childhood T-lineage acute lymphoblastic leukemia. *Blood*, **91**, 735–46.

Wetzler, M., Dodge, R. K., Mrozek, K., *et al.* (1999). Prospective karyotype analysis in adult acute lymphoblastic leukemia: the Cancer and Leukemia Group B experience. *Blood*, **93**, 3983–93.

9

Chronic myeloproliferative disorders and systemic mastocytosis

Introduction

The chronic myeloproliferative disorders (CMPD) are a clinically heterogeneous group of clonal proliferations of stem cell origin characterized, at least initially, by marrow hypercellularity with varying degrees of marrow fibrosis and an increase in the production of one or more terminally differentiated cell types (George & Arber, 2003). These differentiated elements may accumulate in the marrow, in peripheral blood, and in other organs (e.g., spleen). All types of CMPD have a variable tendency to undergo disease progression that may terminate in bone marrow failure due to myelofibrosis or in transformation to an acute leukemic phase, occasionally preceded by a brief myelodysplastic phase. In CMPD, a definite diagnosis usually cannot be made by morphologic examination alone (Anastasi & Vardiman, 2000). The evaluation of bone marrow histology, however, holds an important role in confirming the diagnosis and excluding unsuspected pathology. Expert opinion should be sought if bone marrow histology is to be used as a major diagnostic criterion, since the changes which are specifically associated with the various subtypes of CMPD (see later) are often subtle and difficult to recognize in morphologically less-than-optimal processed samples. This greatly reduces the value of bone marrow histopathology in inexperienced hands (Pearson, 2001).

Classification of these disorders benefits from the integration of morphologic features with clinical, hematologic, and cytogenetic findings (Harris et al., 1999). Of major importance is the presence or absence of the Philadelphia chromosome (BCR/ABL or translocation 9;22), the defining feature of chronic myelogenous leukemia (CML). Essential thrombocythemia (ET), polycythemia vera (PV), and chronic idiopathic myelofibrosis (CIMF) constitute the classical group of BCR/ABL-negative chronic myeloproliferative disorders. Other disorders that will be discussed include chronic neutrophilic leukemia, chronic eosinophilic leukemia/hypereosinophilic syndrome, and systemic mastocytosis.

Chronic myelogenous leukemia

Chronic myelogenous leukemia (CML), formerly referred to as chronic myeloid leukemia or chronic granulocytic leukemia, is the most common CMPD. It can occur at any age, although most cases are seen between 45 and 50 years. The M : F ratio is 1.3 : 1. It is defined by the consistent presence of t(9;22)(q34;q11), also termed the Philadelphia chromosome (Ph[1]), a translocation which causes a BCR/ABL rearrangement (Fig. 9.1). This translocation most commonly produces a fusion protein, termed p210, with increased tyrosine kinase activity. In contrast is the 9;22 translocation of acute leukemias, which is more commonly, but not exclusively, associated with a p190 BCR/ABL fusion protein (Melo, 1996).

CML is a clonal disorder of a multipotent hematopoietic progenitor cell, which is capable of undergoing terminal differentiation but is unresponsive to mechanisms which can normally regulate hematopoietic proliferation. This causes an overproduction of predominantly mature granulocytic cells, which accumulate in the marrow, peripheral blood, and other organs. The granulocytic cells account for most of the proliferation seen in CML, although multiple cell lines demonstrate the Ph[1] chromosome, a finding which is consistent with their derivation from a common clonogenic progenitor.

The peripheral blood examination typically shows a markedly elevated WBC (usually $> 50 \times 10^9/L$) with a preponderance of neutrophils. Also present is a variable number of myeloid precursors in various stages of maturation roughly similar in proportion to their relative

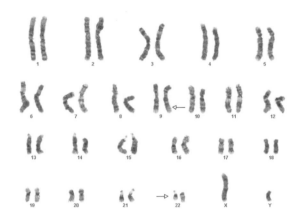

Figure 9.1. Karyotype of chronic myelogenous leukemia (CML), illustrating the derivative chromosome 9;22 (Philadelphia chromosome).

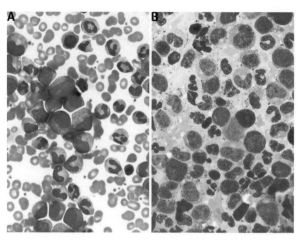

Figure 9.2. Chronic myelogenous leukemia. (A) Peripheral blood smear, showing neutrophilia and circulating granulocyte precursors, mostly myelocytes and metamyelocytes; no blasts are seen. Typically, basophils are increased. (B) Bone marrow aspirate smear obtained from a patient with chronic myelogenous leukemia. Note that the M : E ratio is increased to >10 : 1. Eosinophilic precursors and mature eosinophils are a frequent finding.

frequency in normal bone marrow; blasts are less than 5% and promyelocytes less than 10% of the WBC (Fig. 9.2). Myelocytes are the most numerous myeloid precursors seen in the blood in the chronic phase of CML. Basophils and eosinophils are increased in most cases, with basophilia being most specific for CML. While the absolute number of monocytes may be frequently increased above 1×10^9/L, a relative monocytopenia (<3% of the WBC) is usually observed. Dysplastic features in the granulocytic series are minimal or absent in stable-phase CML. Abnormal basophils that are poorly granulated may be seen. One-third of patients show thrombocytosis; most patients have platelet counts within a normal range. Mild normochromic normocytic anemia is not uncommon. Other characteristic findings include a decreased score for leukocyte alkaline phosphatase (LAP), and elevated levels of lactic dehydrogenase and vitamin B_{12}.

The bone marrow aspirate frequently does not show any fragments but instead shows dense sheets of myeloid cells. The myeloid-to-erythroid ratio is virtually always greater than 10 : 1 in untreated CML, with a mean value of 25 : 1 (normal range 2 : 1 to 5 : 1) (Fig. 9.2). Bone marrow biopsy shows a cellularity approaching 100% in untreated cases with prominent granulocytic hyperplasia. Marrow eosinophils may be substantially increased in some patients. In most cases of CML, the paratrabecular areas show prominent areas of immature myeloid precursors, with more mature forms situated in the intertrabecular areas (Fig. 9.3). Megakaryocytes are increased in number, with a large proportion of small hypolobated forms in clusters and only occasional large bizarre

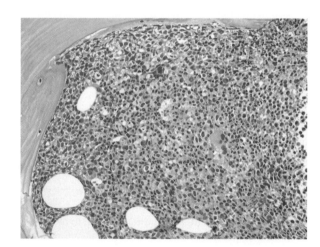

Figure 9.3. Core biopsy of chronic myelogenous leukemia with expansion and layering of the bone trabeculae with immature myeloid elements, the so-called "myeloid bulge."

multilobated forms (Fig. 9.4). True micromegakaryocytes (see Table 7.4) are less common and comprise less than 10% of total megakaryocytopoiesis in CML. Mild reticulin fibrosis ($\leq$1+) is usually observed.

Pseudo-Gaucher histiocytes as well as ceroid-laden (sea-blue) histiocytes are commonly found in CML, reportedly present in 37% to 70% of the cases. The pseudo-Gaucher

Table 9.1. Criteria and findings compatible with classifying the phases of CML.

Chronic phase
   No significant symptoms (after treatment)
   None of the features of accelerated phase or blastic phase
Accelerated phase[a]
   WBC count difficult to control with conventional chemotherapy
   Rapid doubling of WBC count (<5 days)
   Peripheral blood basophils $\geq$20%
   Presence of significant dysgranulopoiesis
   10–19% blasts in peripheral blood or marrow
   $\geq$20% blasts plus promyelocytes in peripheral blood or marrow
   $\geq$20% basophils plus eosinophils in peripheral blood or marrow
   Anemia or thrombocytopenia unresponsive to conventional therapies
   Persistent thrombocytosis ($\geq$1000 $\times$ 10^9/L)
   Additional chromosome changes
   Increasing splenomegaly
   Development of myeloid sarcoma or myelofibrosis
Blastic phase
   $\geq$20% blasts in peripheral blood or marrow
   $\geq$30% blasts plus promyelocytes in peripheral blood or marrow

[a] Any one of these findings is considered adequate by at least one system to fulfill criteria for accelerated phase.

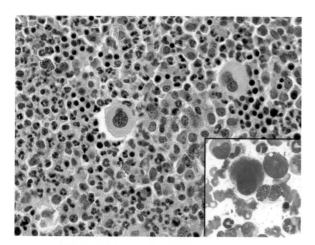

Figure 9.4. Core biopsy of chronic myelogenous leukemia showing "dwarf" megakaryocytes in a background of increased neutrophils and eosinophils. (*Inset*) Bone marrow aspirate smear showing a dwarf megakaryocyte with small nucleus and scanty, mature (granular) cytoplasm.

histiocytes have abundant fibrillar birefringent cytoplasms loaded with cell membrane debris, and have been associated with a more favorable outcome in the cohort of patients receiving chemotherapy. Pseudo-Gaucher cells can be found in the marrow for up to 12 months following

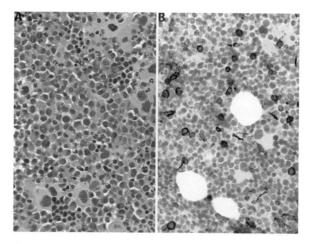

Figure 9.5. Accelerated-phase chronic myelogenous leukemia. (A) Core biopsy showing an increase in immature elements, particularly promyelocytes and blasts, which are difficult to identify on H&E-stained sections. (B) Same case showing increased numbers of CD34-positive blasts.

transplantation. Since these cells can carry the *BCR/ABL* fusion product, but are terminally differentiated cells, their presence may be one cause of persistent PCR positivity early after transplantation that is not predictive of disease relapse (Anastasi *et al.*, 1998).

CML is a biphasic or triphasic disease, i.e., the initial chronic phase, which is essentially defined by the lack of features seen in the more aggressive phases, either changes to an acute blastic phase or, more commonly, evolves into an accelerated phase that later progresses to a blastic phase. The phases of CML have been separated according to various and often poorly consistent criteria. The most commonly used criteria for a diagnosis of accelerated phase require the presence of 10% or more blasts (or 20% of blasts plus promyelocytes) in the peripheral blood or bone marrow. Other criteria for accelerated phase include the development of myelofibrosis, acquisition of additional chromosome abnormalities, marked elevation of the number of blood basophils to $\geq$20% of the WBC, severe granulocytic dysplasia. An increase in the LAP score may also herald an accelerated phase. A complete list is provided in Table 9.1. Bone marrow biopsy is particularly important in identifying the aggressive phases of the disease. The histologic hallmark of accelerated CML is the presence of abnormal aggregation and increased number of blasts and promyelocytes in the marrow (Fig. 9.5). Blasts and promyelocytes frequently form thick layers at the bony trabecular surfaces. Reticulin staining is useful to document the development of significant fibrosis, which is an indication of accelerated disease. The progenitor cell associated-antigen

CD34 is expressed by the blasts in CML (Guyotat *et al.*, 1990; Banavali *et al.*, 1991; Khalidi *et al.*, 1998). CD34 immunostaining can, therefore, be used to facilitate the recognition and to quantitate the number of blasts in CML (Fig. 9.5). In chronic phase CML, CD34-positive cells are seen as rare, isolated cells surrounded by maturing marrow elements. In cases of accelerated-phase CML, the CD34-positive cells are diffusely increased and/or arranged into cell clusters (Orazi *et al.*, 1994; Orazi, 1995).

Detailed immunophenotyping studies are usually necessary to define the nature of the blast cell population in the blastic phase of CML. CD34 is expressed in blasts in 70% or more of the cases of blastic transformation (Khalidi *et al.*, 1998). In up to 70% of the cases myeloblastic transformation is observed (Orazi *et al.*, 1994). In these cases the blast cells show positivity with CD13, CD33, and myeloperoxidase. Lymphoblastic transformation accounts for 15–30% of the cases. Most of these cases show blast cells positive with TdT, CD19, CD79a, and CD10, a precursor B-cell phenotype. However, a high frequency of mixed-lineage phenotype in "lymphoid" blasts has been observed (Khalidi *et al.*, 1998). This most often involves the co-expression on the same cell of precursor B-cell markers (CD19, CD10) and myeloid-associated markers (CD13, CD33, CD61, myeloperoxidase). The frequent lineage infidelity of the blast cells in the blast phase of CML seems to be related to the stem cell origin of this disorder. Such lineage infidelity, however, makes classification of many cases difficult and the significance of, and criteria for, biphenotypic blast crisis of CML is yet to be determined. Cases with a lymphoid immunophenotype, regardless of the co-expression of myeloid markers, have an improved survival and are probably best classified as having lymphoid blast transformation (Cervantes *et al.*, 1998). Megakaryoblastic and other less common subtypes of acute leukemic transformation account for the remaining 5–10% of the cases. Megakaryoblastic transformation often lacks a readable aspirate due to the presence of severe marrow myelofibrosis. In these cases, bone marrow biopsy immunostaining with CD61 and/or factor VIII is particularly useful to confirm the megakaryocytic nature of the blast cells.

Bone marrow biopsy of CML patients treated with α-interferon may appear completely normal (Facchetti *et al.*, 1997). However, the normal morphology does not necessarily correlate with the presence of cytogenetic remission, which occurs only in ≤20% of the IFN-treated patients, and repeated karyotypic and/or *BCR/ABL* analysis is still indicated.

Variability in CML disease phenotype may be due to protein sequences encoded by the translocation partner,

BCR. Different variants have been described in association with the *BCR/ABL* oncoproteins other than p210(*BCR/ABL*). The two most common variants are p190(*BCR/ABL*) and p230(*BCR/ABL*) (Barnes & Melo, 2002).

CML expressing p190(*BCR/ABL*) is relatively rare. From a review of the literature, it may be grouped into two categories: approximately half of the patients exhibited prominent monocytosis and intermediate hematological phenotype between CML, and chronic myelomonocytic leukemia, and the remaining patients showed no monocytosis.

Recently, CML expressing p230(*BCR/ABL*), a less aggressive variant of CML associated with a proliferation of mature neutrophils, has been reported. This variant is termed neutrophilic CML. Although neutrophilic CML morphologically resemble chronic neutrophilic leukemia, the presence of the Ph[1] chromosome associated with a variant *BCR/ABL* translocation producing a 230 kd fusion protein allows for the correct identification of these cases and their inclusion within the spectrum of CML (Pane *et al.*, 1996).

Cases formerly considered to represent Philadelphia chromosome-negative CML on the basis of conventional cytogenetics are often positive for *BCR/ABL* rearrangement when tested by molecular techniques (so called cryptic *BCR/ABL*). These cases should be classified as CML. Rare true Ph[1]-negative cases (cytogenetics plus *BCR/ABL*-negative) are, at present, reclassified as atypical CML or chronic myelomonocytic leukemia within the newly designated group of myelodysplastic/myeloproliferative disorders (described in Chapter 10).

Chronic neutrophilic leukemia

Chronic neutrophilic leukemia (CNL) is an extraordinarily rare type of myeloproliferative disorder observed in elderly patients. It should be distinguished from CML, the neutrophilic variant of CML (CML-N), and chronic myelomonocytic leukemia (CMML). CNL is characterized by the presence of persistent neutrophilic leukocytosis without accompanying immature neutrophilic forms (usually more than 20×10^9/L), lack of basophilia, increased leukocyte alkaline phosphatase activity, and anatomic evidence of organ infiltration by granulocytes, granulocytes with immature forms, and/or myeloid metaplasia (Jaffe *et al.*, 2001). The Philadelphia chromosome and the *BCR/ABL* fusion gene are absent. The peripheral blood, marrow aspirate, and biopsy show significant neutrophilic hyperplasia. The lack of monocytosis in the peripheral blood and absence of significant dysplastic changes in the bone marrow are features which help in distinguishing CNL from the myelodysplastic/myeloproliferative disorders, chronic myelomonocytic leukemia, and atypical CML in particular. Patients with CNL may demonstrate a clonal evolution during the course of the disease, and blastic transformation has been reported. CNL patients initially respond to therapy with hydroxyurea with control of leukocytosis and reduction in splenomegaly. However, most patients eventually become refractory to treatment, manifesting progressive neutrophilia without blastic transformation. The clinical course is heterogeneous, with a definite risk of death from either blastic transformation or progressive neutrophilic leukocytosis. Most patients have a normal karyotype. Reported abnormalities may include +8, +9, and del(20q) (Orazi *et al.*, 1989). Cases of neutrophilic CML are separated by the presence of Ph[1] chromosome associated with a variant p230 (*BCR/ABL*) fusion protein.

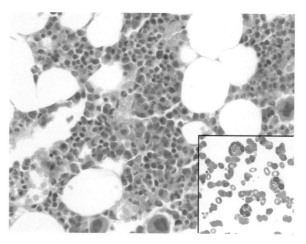

Figure 9.6. Chronic eosinophilic leukemia (CEL). Note the large increase in eosinophilic precursors in the bone marrow. (*Inset*) Peripheral blood smear showing abnormal, hyperlobulated eosinophils.

Chronic eosinophilic leukemia/ hypereosinophilic syndrome

Chronic eosinophilic leukemia (CEL) and idiopathic hypereosinophilic syndrome (HES) are rare and poorly defined entities which may present with a variety of symptoms including weight loss, sweats, skin rashes, and cardiac abnormalities (Bain, 1996). The cardiac damage is probably due to the toxic effects on the endomyocardium exerted by released cationic proteins present in the eosinophilic granules. Splenomegaly and hepatosplenomegaly are found in 40–80% of the patients. The peripheral blood shows significant eosinophilia (defined as $>1.5 \times 10^9$/L eosinophils) present for more than six months. Neutrophilia and basophilia may accompany the eosinophilia. Anemia and thrombocytopenia may be observed in a proportion of the patients. A proportion of the eosinophils show cytoplasmic vacuolization and/or degranulation. The bone marrow is hypercellular with an increased myeloid-to-erythroid ratio, significant eosinophilia, and a variable amount of reticulin fibrosis (Fig. 9.6). Macrophages with Charcot–Leyden granules can be observed.

CEL/HES must also be distinguished from other causes of eosinophilia such as parasite infections and allergies, and the elevation of eosinophils seen in patients with various hematologic and non-hematologic malignancies.

Distinction between the two conditions of CEL and HES relies on a combination of morphologic and cytogenetic findings. In cases of CEL, an increased proportion of blasts and abnormal maturing eosinophilic precursors is noted. In HES, eosinophilia may be marked, but immature and dysplastic cells are usually absent and cytogenetic abnormalities are absent. Cytogenetic studies are often necessary to confirm the presence of clonality, to exclude the presence of *BCR/ABL*, and therefore confirm a diagnosis of CEL. Once it is determined that the proliferation of eosinophils is clonal, idiopathic hypereosinophilic syndrome is probably not an appropriate term to define a case and should be dropped. Cases of myelodysplastic syndrome with eosinophilia as well as eosinophilic-rich variants of CML have been reported (see Chapter 7). In these cases, however, the eosinophilia is largely restricted to the bone marrow, while the peripheral blood more often shows pancytopenia in the former condition and neutrophilia in the latter. Rare cases of eosinophilic CMML have also been reported (see Chapter 10).

A variety of cytogenetic abnormalities are reported in patients with CEL; the commonest are +8, i(17q), and t(5;12)(q33;p13) (Berkowicz *et al.*, 1991; Bain, 1996). The latter abnormality, however, has also been reported in cases of MDS and CMML with eosinophilia. Marked eosinophilia can also occur in a group of myeloproliferative syndromes associated with translocations involving the chromosome band 8p11 (Macdonald *et al.*, 1995; Reiter *et al.*, 1998). These disorders are characterized by a chronic myelogenous leukemia-like myeloid hyperplasia and a strikingly high incidence of non-Hodgkin lymphoma, mostly of T-lymphoblastic subtype (Macdonald *et al.*, 1995). After a short chronic phase of 6 to 9 months, they rapidly transform into an AML. The median survival time is less than 12 months. A subset of cases of CEL/HES respond to the tyrosine kinase inhibitor, imatinib mesylate (Cools *et al.*, 2003).

Chronic basophilic leukemia

This entity is extraordinarily rare (Pardanani *et al.*, 2003a). There have only been a few literature reports, but it does seem to be a real clinical entity. As expected, it is a neoplastic proliferation of basophils. They can have dysplastic morphology. The differential diagnosis is most important, because of its rarity. First and foremost, CML must be ruled out. Any case associated with an increased number of basophils and *BCR/ABL* should be considered CML. There are rare chronic infections and allergic conditions that can cause peripheral blood basophilia; its degree is typically minimal and the basophils do not display dysplastic features.

Chronic idiopathic myelofibrosis with myeloid metaplasia

Chronic idiopathic myelofibrosis (CIMF) (formerly referred to as agnogenic myeloid metaplasia, primary idiopathic myelofibrosis, myelosclerosis) is a clonal stem cell disease characterized by progressive marrow failure associated with variable degrees of bone marrow fibrosis, splenomegaly, and extramedullary hematopoiesis (Thiele *et al.*, 1996; Manoharan, 1998; Barosi *et al.*, 1999). It usually appears in middle-aged to elderly individuals, and only rarely in younger people. There is an approximately equal incidence of CIMF in males and females. The peripheral blood smear in advanced stages of the disease shows teardrop red blood cells associated with a leukoerythroblastic picture characterized by the presence of normoblasts and myeloid precursors that include myelocytes and metamyelocytes. A variable number of myeloblasts is observed. In most cases, these cells represent <5% of the WBC; however, a blast count of up to 10% (in the absence of blastic transformation) may be observed. Megathrombocytes (or giant platelets, defined as larger than a red blood cell) and bare megakaryocytic nuclei are frequently observed. Teardrop erythrocytes have been noted to decrease in number following splenectomy or institution of chemotherapy. In approximately 60% of patients, the hemoglobin level drops to 10g/dL. Leukopenia is seen in 13–25% of patients, while leukocytosis is seen in one-third. In 31% of patients, thrombocytopenia is observed; thrombocytosis is seen in 12%. Those cases may be clinically indistinguishable from essential throm-

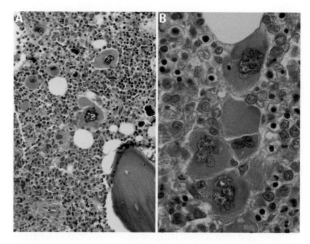

Figure 9.7. Chronic idiopathic myelofibrosis (CIMF). (A) Note the hypercellular marrow with granulocytic and megakaryocytic hyperplasia. (B) High magnification of the core biopsy showing a tight cluster of highly pleomorphic, large megakaryocytes displaying abnormal chromatin clumping and "cloud"-shaped nuclei.

bocythemia (ET). The bone marrow is rarely aspirable. A bone marrow biopsy is necessary in all cases to assess the amount of hematopoietic tissue and the degree of marrow fibrosis.

In the early stages of the disease, the marrow biopsy may show hypercellular marrow with an increased myeloid-to-erythroid ratio, and little or no fibrosis (prefibrotic phase) (Thiele *et al.*, 1999). However, this early phase is often undocumented, and by the time of the initial biopsy most patients show already a more advanced picture characterized by patchiness of the hematopoietic cellularity with alternately cellular (non-fibrotic) and less cellular (fibrotic) areas (Fig. 9.7). It is particularly important to separate cases of early CIMF with thrombocytosis (not uncommon) from the more benign ET. Even in these early cases of CIMF, however, abnormal megakaryopoiesis is always present, and if close attention is paid to the cytologic and histotopographic characteristics of these cells, as seen in bone marrow biopsies (Fig. 9.7), distinction from other types of myeloproliferative disorder, ET in particular, can be reliably achieved (Thiele *et al.*, 2000). In CIMF, the megakaryocytes are predominantly large, atypical, with abnormally clumped chromatin with cloud-like or balloon-shaped lobulation of megakaryocytic nuclei (Fig. 9.7). These megakaryocytic abnormalities are not seen in other types of CMPDs at diagnosis and during follow-up (Thiele & Kvasnicka, 2000). In addition, "tight" clusters of megakaryocytes, with little or no space between the megakaryocytes,

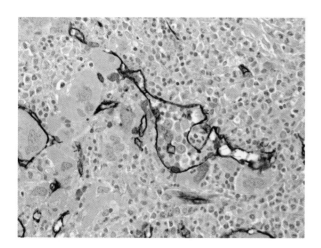

Figure 9.8. Dilated sinusoids immunostained by CD34, displaying intravascular hematopoiesis. This is a characteristic finding in advanced-stage CIMF.

is considered to be more characteristic of CIMF than other CMPDs. The megakaryocytes are surrounded by granulocytic cells more often than by erythroblasts.

The advanced stage of the disease is characterized by significant fibrosis (88% ≥2+, 67% ≥3+ in one study) and myeloid metaplasia causing splenomegaly. Clusters of atypical megakaryocytes are particularly prominent in more markedly fibrotic areas. Distended marrow sinusoids containing intravascular hematopoietic cells and megakaryocytes (Fig. 9.8) are characteristic findings observed in these advanced cases (Wolf *et al.*, 1988). Significant sclerosis of bone trabeculae also occurs in many patients. Lymphoid aggregates predominantly composed of reactive T lymphocytes are also seen in many CIMF patients. Myeloid metaplasia (extramedullary hematopoiesis) can occur in a variety of tissue sites. Common sites of involvement include spleen, liver, lungs, kidneys, and gastrointestinal tract.

In the early phases of CIMF, the number of CD34-positive cells seen in the bone marrow is usually within normal limits. While the disease progresses, their number decreases. This parallels their egression from the marrow into the blood and to the myeloid metaplasia-prone organs (e.g., spleen). However, in some cases of advanced-stage CIMF, CD34-positive cells may actually increase, paralleling the increased number of myeloblasts. Between 10% and 20% of patients with CIMF transform to AML. In most of these cases, however, the findings on the marrow biopsy remain unchanged since the acute transformation is seen at least initially in extramedullary sites (e.g., spleen). In CIMF and cases of post-polycythemic myeloid metaplasia (see

polycythemia vera, below) biopsies, immunostaining with CD34, vWF, and CD31 can be used to facilitate the detection of intravascular hematopoiesis, a characteristic and diagnostically useful finding in these disorders. The presence of increased angiogenesis in CIMF patients has been found to correlate with the degree of splenomegaly and aggressive clinical course (Mesa *et al.*, 2000). No correlation was found between the degree of angiogenesis and amount of reticulin fibrosis (Mesa *et al.*, 2000; Orazi *et al.*, 2001).

The differential diagnosis of CIMF may occasionally be complicated since a number of other disorders may lead to a similar clinical picture. Especially complicated may be the distinction with other types of myeloproliferative disorders and myelodysplastic syndromes. A variant of myelodysplastic syndrome, myelodysplastic syndrome with fibrosis (MDS-f; see Chapter 7), in particular, can be difficult to separate from CIMF. MDS-f, however, is characterized by reticulocytopenia, often severe dysgranulopoieis, predominance in the marrow of hypolobated megakaryocytes and micromegakaryocytes, and the frequent presence of ALIP easily identified by CD34 immunostaining. None of these features is typically seen in CIMF. Unlike patients with CIMF, patients with MDS-f do not have hepatic or splenic enlargement extending beyond 30 mm below the costal margin.

Myelofibrosis can occur as a late event in patients with other myeloproliferative disorders, especially polycythemia vera (e.g., post-polycythemic myeloid metaplasia) and CML, and, rarely, essential thrombocytopenia. The morphologic features in these late stages can be identical to CIMF. In these conditions, CML and polycythemia vera in particular, the development of marrow fibrosis may herald the onset of accelerated phase or blastic transformation.

Immunohistochemistry can also be useful to rule out metastatic carcinoma when suspicious cells are observed within a fibrotic marrow (see Chapter 13). Staining with vWF, CD61, CD42b, or other platelet-reactive antibodies can also be useful to demonstrate the presence of megakaryoblasts in cases of acute myelofibrosis and acute megakaryoblastic leukemia, and to separate those from CIMF.

The diagnostic criteria proposed by an Italian consensus group (Barosi *et al.*, 1999) identify two "necessary" criteria: diffuse bone marrow fibrosis and absence of the Philadelphia chromosome (or *BCR/ABL* rearrangement), and six "optional" criteria: splenomegaly of any grade; anisopoikilocytosis with teardrop erythrocytes; the presence of circulating immature myeloid cells; the presence of circulating erythroblasts; the presence of clusters of megakaryoblasts and anomalous megakaryocytes in bone marrow sections; and myeloid metaplasia. Recently, a consensus conference

Table 9.2. Consensus on the grading of myelofibrosis (MF) in CIMF based on the European Consensus Conference for grading of marrow fibrosis and assessment of cellularity, Palermo, Italy, October 2004.

Grading	Description[a]
MF-0	Scattered linear reticulin with no intersections (crossovers) corresponding to normal BM
MF-1	Loose network of reticulin with many intersections, especially in perivascular areas
MF-2	Diffuse and dense increase in reticulin with extensive intersections, occasionally with only focal bundles of collagen and/or focal osteosclerosis
MF-3	Diffuse and dense increase in reticulin with extensive intersections with coarse bundles of collagen, often associated with significant osteosclerosis

[a] Fiber density should be assessed in hematopoietic (cellular) areas.
Adapted from Thiele *et al.*, 2005

has attempted to standardize the assessment of myelofibrosis and cellularity in CIMF (Thiele *et al.*, 2005). The proposed new grading system for myelofibrosis is shown in Table 9.2. A reliable definition of the disease as CIMF is achieved when the two necessary criteria are fulfilled, plus any other two criteria when splenomegaly is present or any four when splenomegaly is absent.

Cytogenetic analysis is frequently performed to rule out the presence of the Ph[1] chromosome. In CIMF, karyotypic abnormalities are reported in approximately 35–60% of the patients. The most common abnormalities found in these cases include deletion of 1q, 20q, 13q, and acquired trisomy 8, 9, 21, or 21p+ (Reilly *et al.*, 1997).

Median survival is 40 to 65 months from diagnosis (Table 9.3). The most frequent causes of death in CIMF patients are marrow failure (22%), including anemia, infections, and hemorrhage; transformation to AML (up to 15–20% of cases); and portal hypertension related to massive splenomegaly (Dupriez *et al.*, 1996).

CIMF is very rare in children (Hamazaki & Mugishima, 1981; Wang *et al.*, 1990). A review of 15 cases of myelofibrosis in children collected from the literature showed a mean age of 2 years and 9 months with most patients being less than 2 years of age. The survival in these cases was short (less than 8 months). However, several recent studies of cases

Table 9.3. Scoring system for CIMF.

Risk factors
  Hgb < 10 g/dL
  WBC < 4 ×10^9/L
  WBC > 30 ×10^9/L
Prognosis
  (a) No risk factors: median survival 93 months
  (b) 1 risk factor: median survival 26 months
  (c) 2 risk factors: median survival 13 months

Adapted from Dupriez *et al.*, 1996

of pediatric idiopathic myelofibrosis have challenged these conclusions by showing a different clinical course in infants from adults, with lack of significant organomegaly and prolonged spontaneous remissions in the former group (Altura *et al.*, 2000). The reported occurrence of the disease in two siblings is suggestive of an autosomal recessive mode of inheritance for some of the pediatric cases (Sekhar *et al.*, 1996).

Polycythemia vera

Polycythemia vera (PV) is a clonal progressive myeloproliferative disorder characterized by an absolute increase in red cell mass, often with leukocytosis, thrombocytosis, and variable splenomegaly (Murphy, 1999; Pearson, 2001). PV usually occurs in elderly patients, with a male predominance. Two phases of the disease occur. The first phase, known as the erythrocytotic (proliferative) phase, is a relatively indolent disease with median survival rates of 10–15 years. The second phase, known as post-polycythemic myeloid metaplasia or spent phase, is an aggressive end-stage disease with median survival of less than 2.5 years.

The peripheral blood in the erythrocytotic phase characteristically shows increased hemoglobin and hematocrit; however, these levels may be decreased if iron deficiency has occurred. If the hematocrit exceeds 60%, an elevated RBC volume is almost always seen. The erythrocytes may show normal cytology or changes compatible with iron deficiency anemia. Rarely, circulating normoblasts are seen. The WBC count is only moderately increased with a left-shifted granulocytosis. The basophil count may be slightly elevated, but is typically lower than seen in CML. Platelet count may exceed 600 × 10^9/L, a finding which may suggest a possible diagnosis of essential thrombocythemia. In its initial, prodromic stages, PV can be easily confused with ET, particularly since both hematocrit and RBC volume may not be significantly increased (Thiele & Kvasnicka, 2005).

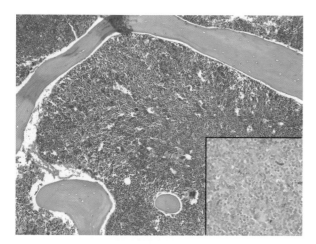

Figure 9.9. Polycythemia vera (PV). Core biopsy showing a hypercellular bone marrow, with an increase in the erythroid precursors and megakaryocytes. (*Inset*) Iron stain – which is negative – a finding typical of PV.

The bone marrow in patients with PV is usually moderately hypercellular with trilineage hyperplasia (Fig. 9.9). Erythropoiesis, in contrast with some other chronic myeloproliferative disorders, may be predominant. Megakaryocytes are increased in number and are highly pleomorphic; those of large or giant size show hyperlobulated nuclei lacking significant dysplastic features; overall, megakaryocytes seen in PV are more similar to those seen in essential thrombocythemia than the ones in CIMF. They appear dispersed or form loose clusters around marrow sinusoids or lie close to the bony trabeculae. Often they are surrounded by maturing erythroid cells. The slightly increased cellularity and the presence of pleomorphic megakaryocytes help in distinguishing initial stages of PV (see above) from ET, which lacks those features (Thiele & Kvasnicka, 2005). Of the three proliferating cell lines, granulopoiesis is often the least conspicuous. Marrow fibrosis is usually only minimal in this phase of the disease. Splenomegaly in the erythrocytotic phase of PV is primarily due to splenic red pulp congestion and is usually of modest degree (Wolf *et al.*, 1988). Only 6% of the PV patients show presence of stainable iron (Thiele & Kvasnicka, 2005) (Fig. 9.9).

The spent phase of PV, also termed post-polycythemic myeloid metaplasia (PPMM), is a late stage of the disorder, usually seen after 8–10 years' latency. The spent phase is associated with the development of progressive marrow fibrosis, decreased erythropoiesis and overall marrow cellularity, and peripheral blood changes similar or identical to those observed in CIMF. Only in this phase of

PV does splenomegaly become prominent. Splenic myeloid metaplasia is not a feature of uncomplicated polycythemia vera, and its presence indicates progression to the spent phase (Wolf *et al.*, 1988). In the spent phase of PV, the marrow histology findings are indistinguishable from those seen in the advanced stages of CIMF and the differentiation of these two conditions may not be possible without a documented previous history of PV.

Because of the non-specific morphologic findings and clinical overlap between PV and other myeloproliferative and reactive conditions, detailed diagnostic criteria are described for this disorder (Table 9.4). A diagnosis of PV is established if three major criteria are present, or if two major criteria (increased RBC mass and normal arterial oxygen saturation) and two minor criteria are met. Of other parameters that can be used to confirm a diagnosis of polycythemia vera, the most useful is the measurement of serum erythropoietin level. PV requires evidence of an erythropoietin-independent increase in red blood cell mass (low erythropoietin levels). The documentation of spontaneous formation of erythroid cell colonies in cell culture has also been proposed as a useful technique to detect very early stages of the disease in which the standard diagnostic tests (e.g., red blood cell mass analysis) are still within normal limits. RBC mass in particular may be "falsely" decreased in PV patients who also have iron deficiency, and the analysis may have to be repeated after iron supplement therapy for an accurate diagnostic result. Reactive or secondary polycythemia must also be excluded and it may be related to smoking, lung and kidney diseases, erythropoietin-producing tumors (kidney, liver, brain), and exogenous administration of erythropoietin. Among the rare congenital conditions causing erythropoietin production, familial secondary polycythemias due to high oxygen affinity hemoglobin mutants are not infrequent and have been well delineated in terms of molecular pathophysiology and phenotype during the last three decades. Very rare secondary familial polycythemias due to 2,3-biphosphoglycerate (2,3-BPG, previously known as 2,3-DPG) deficiency also occur.

Familial and congenital polycythemias with increased erythropoietin concentration and normal arterial oxygen saturation and oxygen dissociation kinetics represent an intriguing group of disorders wherein the molecular lesions remain obscure (Prchal, 2001). These conditions need to be distinguished from the so-called primary familial and congenital polycythemia (PFCP or familial erythrocytosis), a rare condition of autosomal dominant inheritance or sporadic occurrence which is the result of a congenital defect in the erythropoietin receptor and is associated with normal oxygen saturation and normal erythropoietin levels

Table 9.4. Criteria for the diagnosis of polycythemia vera (PVSG, modified PVSG, and WHO).

	PVSG	Modified PVSG	WHO
Major criteria			
A1	Red blood cell mass of >36 mL/kg in males or >32 mL/kg in females	Red cell mass >25% above mean normal value	Red cell mass >25% above mean normal value, or increased Hgb >18.5 g/dL in males, >16.5 g/dL in females
A2	Arterial oxygen saturation of >92%	Absence of secondary erythrocytosis	Absence of secondary erythrocytosis
A3	Splenomegaly on palpation	Splenomegaly on palpation	Splenomegaly on palpation
A4	—	Clonality marker, e.g. abnormal marrow karyotype	Clonal evidence other than Ph^1+ or *BCR/ABL*
A5	—	—	Spontaneous EEC
Minor criteria			
B1	Thrombocytosis/platelet count of >400 × 10^9/L	Platelets >400 × 10^9/L	Platelets >400 × 10^9/L
B2	White blood cell count of >12 × 10^9/L with no fever or infection	Leukocytes >12 × 10^9/L	Leukocytes >12 × 10^9/L
B3	Elevated neutrophil alkaline phosphatase level of >100	Splenomegaly on ultrasound	Bone marrow biopsy with typical PV picture
B4	—	Spontaneous EEC or low serum EPO	Low serum EPO
Diagnosis of PV			
	A1 + A2 + A3	A1 + A2 + A3 or A4	A1 + A2 + any other from A
	A1 + A2 + two from B	A1 + A2 + two from B	A1 + A2 + two from B

PVSG, Polycythemia Vera Study Group; EEC, endogenous erythroid colony formation; EPO, erythropoietin

(Prchal, 2001). Various mutations have been described in these cases.

Secondary polycythemia usually lacks the increased marrow cellularity secondary to the presence of trilineage hyperplasia (e.g., subcortical bioptic areas are hypocellular, in contrast with what is seen in true PV), the increased reticulin content, and above all the increased megakaryopoiesis characterized by clusters of pleomorphic, often large megakaryocytes with hyperlobulated nuclei, as seen in PV. Additionally, in secondary polycythemia, stainable iron is usually detected. The histopathologic evaluation is of particular value in cases of secondary polycythemia since, in a proportion of these cases, EPO levels may be "falsely" low.

Approximately 10% of PV patients will transform to acute leukemia, typically acute myeloid leukemia, within 15 years from the diagnosis, and up to half within 20 years. Acute leukemia onset may be preceded by a myelodysplastic phase. Rare cases of acute lymphoblastic leukemia have also been reported. The incidence of acute leukemia in patients with PV treated by therapeutic phlebotomies alone is very low, particularly in cases without karyotypic abnormalities at presentation. In contrast, acute leukemia is reported to occur in approximately 10% of patients receiving radioactive phosphorus and 14% of patients receiving alkylating agents, raising the possibility of therapy-related AML/MDS. Non-radiomimetic drugs, hydroxyurea and pipobroman, are also associated with an increased risk of leukemia in PV patients; the risk is estimated to be between 1% and 5.9% with hydroxyurea therapy (Nand *et al.*, 1996). Leukemic transformation in PV often presents as a therapy-related myelodysplastic syndrome that rapidly progresses to overt acute leukemia. Rare cases of Ph^1-positive CML and non-Hodgkin lymphoma, also thought to be therapy-related, have been reported.

Cytogenetic analysis in cases of suspected PV is used to rule out the presence of Ph^1 chromosome. Karyotype abnormalities which are not specific for PV may be detected in up to 50% of PV cases (Dewald & Wright, 1995). A few of the most frequently found non-random anomalies include trisomy 8 and 9, double trisomy 8+9, 20q− and trisomy of part or all of 1q. Other recurring aberrations such as 13q− occur mainly in late stages of PV, in which complex, unstable karyotypes are also commonly found (Tanzer, 1994). Recently, the overexpression of a hematopoietic receptor, polycythemia rubra vera 1 (PRV-1), in patients with PV has been proposed as a novel diagnostic tool. PV patients express significantly higher amounts of PRV-1 than

Table 9.5. Criteria for the diagnosis of essential thrombocythemia.

Platelet count >600 × 10^9/L

No cause of reactive thrombocytosis

Hematocrit <40% or normal cell mass (<36 mL/kg in males and <32 mL/kg in females)

Normal red blood cell mean corpuscular volume, serum ferritin, or marrow iron stain

Collagen fibrosis absent or less than one-third of biopsy area without both splenomegaly and leukoerythroblastic reaction

No cytogenetic or morphologic evidence of myelodysplasia

No Philadelphia chromosome or *BCR/ABL* gene rearrangement

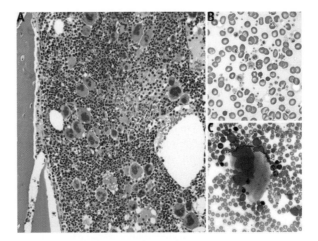

Figure 9.10. Essential thrombocythemia (ET). (A) Core biopsy showing increased number of large megakaryocytes with hyperlobulated nuclei but otherwise devoid of significant dysplasia. The clusters of megakaryocytes in this condition are less tight than those seen in CIMF. Marrow cellularity, myelopoiesis, and erythropoiesis are all within normal limits. (B) Peripheral blood smear showing numerous platelets; atypical forms and giant platelets are noticeable. (C) Bone marrow aspirate smear showing a single hyperlobulated megakaryocyte and unremarkable granulocytes.

healthy controls or patients with secondary erythrocytosis (Pahl, 2003). In addition, decreased expression of the thrombopoietin receptor c-Mp1 and insulin-like growth factor-I hypersensitivity have also been reported. However, prospective studies are necessary to evaluate the usefulness of these markers in a clinical setting, since overlaps between PV and ET have been noted (Thiele & Kvasnicka, 2005).

Essential thrombocythemia

Essential thrombocythemia (ET) is a chronic myeloproliferative disorder characterized by persistent significant thrombocytosis. The age distribution is broad, ranging from adolescent to old patients; most cases are seen in patients older than 50 years. Well-documented cases in young adults and children have been reported. Rare familial forms of ET have been also seen.

The CBC shows a platelet count that is usually above 1000 × 10^9/L; the platelet count must be at least 600 × 10^9/L (Murphy *et al.*, 1997) to fulfill criteria published by the Polycythemia Vera Study Group (PVSG; Table 9.5). The thrombocytosis is usually accompanied by the presence of abnormally large platelets, often aggregated into large platelet clumps (Fig. 9.10). As a reflection of the large platelet size, the mean platelet volume is markedly increased, while the observed high platelet distribution width reflects a wide spectrum of platelet size. Circulating megakaryocyte nuclei and cytoplasmic fragments may be observed in cases of ET. Leukocytosis, when present, is usually mild, does not exceed 30 × 10^9/L, and lacks left-shifted forms or basophilia. Red blood cell morphology is usually unremarkable. The bone marrow is usually normocellular or only slightly hypercellular (hypocellularity is rare) and displays megakaryocytic hyperplasia (Fig. 9.10). The megakaryocytes occur predominantly in loose clus-

ters and tend to be large to giant in size with abundant cytoplasm and hyperlobulated nuclei devoid of dysplastic features. Their median size is larger than those seen in reactive conditions and in CML. Emperipolesis of neutrophils is frequently noted within the megakaryocyte cytoplasm. The myeloid-to-erythroid ratio is close to normal, and marrow fibrosis is minimal or absent. In contrast with PV, stainable iron is identifiable in the marrow in the majority of the ET cases. Increased angiogenesis and prominent intravascular hematopoiesis as seen in CIMF are not usually observed in ET.

The most frequent complication of ET includes thrombotic and hemorrhagic phenomena (Besses *et al.*, 1999). Transformation into acute leukemia, usually AML, is seen in less than 5% of the patients (Mesa *et al.*, 1999). Rare cases show a progression into a "spent" phase similar to that seen in PV patients with post-polycythemic myeloid metaplasia; such progression is, however, uncommon and an alternative diagnosis of CIMF or PV should be first excluded by reviewing the material on the basis of which the original diagnosis of ET was rendered.

The value of ancillary studies in ET is similar to that for other myeloproliferative disorders. Recently, decreased expression of c-Mpl in the megakaryocytes of ET, compared to megakaryocytes of reactive thrombocytosis, has been suggested as a helpful marker of the disease (Mesa *et al.*, 2002). The detection of clonal cytogenetic abnormalities is useful in confirming the neoplastic nature of the process, but most cases do not demonstrate such abnormalities. Although rare Ph[1] chromosome-positive ET cases are described in the literature, it has been proposed that they be considered examples of CML because of a shared propensity to progress to blast crisis (LeBrun *et al.*, 1991).

The differential diagnoses include cases of early-stage polycythemia vera with associated thrombocytosis that might mimic ET (see previous section). Paying close attention to the marrow cellularity and its composition, and to the cytologic characteristics of the megakaryocytes, usually allows separation of these disorders (Thiele & Kvasnicka, 2005). Red cell mass studies, erythropoietin level determination, and/or endogenous erythroid colony formation analysis may also be indicated in such instances.

Essential thrombocythemia has been traditionally considered to be a clonal disorder, although no specific karyotypic abnormalities have been described. Cytogenetic abnormalities are rare, but analysis using X-chromosome inactivation patterns indicates that nearly 50% of evaluable patients have polyclonal myelopoiesis, and this is associated with a lower risk of thrombosis (Harrison *et al.*, 1999). Reduced and/or heterogeneous expression of c-Mpl in bone marrow biopsies may help to distinguish ET from reactive thrombocytosis. Increased expression of PRV-1 (polycythemia rubra vera) messenger RNA in granulocytes may assist in discrimination between polycythemia vera and at least some cases of ET (Gale, 2003). More recently decreased expression of c-Mp1 in megakaryocytes of patients with ET has been shown to be of value in distinguishing hereditary ET from reactive thrombocytosis (Mesa *et al.*, 2002).

Systemic mastocytosis

An increased number of mast cells in the bone marrow can be seen with a variety of hematologic diseases, including chronic lymphoproliferative disorders (e.g., lymphoplasmacytic lymphoma and chronic lymphocytic leukemia), myelodysplastic and myeloproliferative disorders, subtypes of acute myeloid leukemia, aplastic anemia, and autoimmune conditions. Primary mast cell disorders are rare. They are generally classified in four groups (Table 9.6). The systemic forms of the disease are characterized by a generalized infiltration of mast cells involving many organs, most notably the bone marrow, spleen, liver, and lymph nodes; cutaneous involvement may or may not be present. Clinically most patients with systemic mastocy-

Table 9.6. Mast cell diseases: WHO classification.

Cutaneous mastocytosis
Systemic mast cell disease (+/− skin involvement)
Systemic mast cell disease with an associated hematologic disorder (+/− skin involvement)
Mast cell leukemia/sarcoma

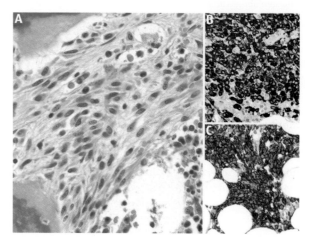

Figure 9.11. Mastocytosis. (A) High magnification showing numerous spindled cells with only faintly granular cytoplasm. (B) Tryptase immunohistochemical stain in mastocytosis. (C) CD117 immunohistochemical stain in mastocytosis.

tosis have severe anemia and bone marrow involvement with the disease (Horny *et al.*, 1997). On X-ray, 70% of patients have skeletal lesions: osteopenia in 44%, multiple osteolytic lesions in 22%, and osteosclerotic lesions in 27% (Huang *et al.*, 1987). A large proportion of patients develop a myeloproliferative disorder, usually unclassifiable. Other patients develop atypical chronic myeloid leukemia, chronic myelomonocytic leukemia (Smith & Lazarchick, 1999), or myelodysplastic syndromes. A small percentage of patients transform into mast cell leukemia (Escribano *et al.*, 1997). Rarely, other types of acute leukemia have also been reported.

In the bone marrow, the characteristic findings in mastocytosis include the presence of multiple nodular, perivascular and/or paratrabecular lesions, composed of pale, frequently spindle-shaped mast cells with oval or reniform nuclei, admixed with a variable number of eosinophils and lymphocytes (Fig. 9.11). Significant fibrosis, often paratrabecular, and thickening of bone with evidence of osseous remodeling are typically observed in proximity of paratrabecular mast cell aggregates.

Due to the presence of fibrosis, the bone marrow aspirate may yield a "false negative" result; however when particles are present in the aspirate material, spindled mast cells are frequently present embedded in the particles. The mast cells may appear poorly granulated, particularly in sclerotic lesions. Hypogranulated spindled mast cells can be mistaken for fibroblasts, and an erroneous diagnosis of myelofibrosis can be made. In contrast to myelofibrosis, however, the sclerotic areas in mast cell disease are devoid of megakaryocytes. Occasionally, the mast cells are polygonal or round and have abundant pale cytoplasm that is only minimally granulated. In this case the mast cells may resemble histiocytes, or the cells of hairy cell leukemia, or monocytoid variants of marginal zone lymphoma.

The lymphocytic hyperplasia seen in marrows involved with systemic mastocytosis may occasionally be so extensive as to mimic a lymphoproliferative disorder. Immunophenotyping with lymphoid reactive antibodies usually shows a mixture of B and T lymphocytes and no evidence of lymphoma.

Sheets of atypical or frankly malignant mast cells may be rarely seen on bone marrow sections. This pattern is usually associated with peripheral blood involvement by mast cells (mast cell leukemia). Mast cell leukemia can follow systemic mastocytosis or occur *de novo*. This disease is associated with a dismal prognosis. No therapies have been proven effective.

On bone marrow biopsy, one can rarely encounter a truly isolated form of mast cell disease. This entity, which corresponds to cases previously termed eosinophilic fibrohistiocytic lesion of bone marrow, is characterized by collections of elongated "fibrohistiocytic" mast cells in association with lymphocytes, eosinophils, and plasma cells. Many investigators consider this lesion a localized form of mastocytosis, which lacks skin involvement, remains confined to the bone marrow, and is incapable of evolving into a generalized form.

Although the diagnosis is traditionally established after staining with Giemsa or toluidine blue, the mast cells can also be immunostained with CD117 and CD68/KP-1 monoclonal antibodies (Li *et al.*, 1996) (Fig. 9.11). Special stain for chloroacetate esterase (CAE), which is frequently used to identify mast cells in extramedullary sites (e.g., skin), is inhibited by nitric acid decalcification and is therefore not used to stain bone marrow biopsies that are so processed. Mast cells are also positive, in most cases, with an antibody to tartrate-resistant acid phosphate (TRAP). Anti-tryptase has been shown to be the most specific marker for the diagnosis of mast cell disorders (Horny *et al.*, 1998; Yang *et al.*, 2000). In cases of malignant mast cell disease, the anti-tryptase antibody can correctly identify a higher proportion

of the malignant mast cells than CAE or Giemsa. Chymase is another recently proposed marker for mast cells (Buckley *et al.*, 1999). The expression of CD25 in mast cells has been reported only in neoplastic mast cells, and has been consistently identified on bone marrow mast cells of patients with systemic mastocytosis and not in reactive conditions (Pardanani *et al.*, 2004). In addition, a mutation of the *c-KIT* gene can be demonstrated in a proportion of patients with systemic mastocytosis (Pardanani *et al.*, 2003b). The mutation seems to be significantly associated with advanced age, an aggressive clinical course, high bone marrow mast cell content, and co-existence of chronic myelomonocytic leukemia or other clonal hematological non-mast cell disease (Horny *et al.*, 2004).

REFERENCES

Altura, R. A., Head, D. R., & Wang, W. C. (2000). Long-term survival of infants with idiopathic myelofibrosis. *British Journal of Haematology*, **109**, 459–62.

Anastasi, J. & Vardiman, J. W. (2000). Chronic myelogenous leukemia and the myeloproliferative disorders. In *Neoplastic Hematopathology*, ed. D. M. Knowles, 2nd edn. Baltimore: Williams & Wilkins, pp. 1745–60.

Anastasi, J., Musvee, T., Roulston, D., Domer, P. H., Larson, R. A., & Vardiman, J. W. (1998). Pseudo-Gaucher histiocytes identified up to 1 year after transplantation for CML are BCR/ABL-positive. *Leukemia*, **12**, 233–7.

Bain, B. J. (1996). Eosinophilic leukaemias and the idiopathic hypereosinophilic syndrome. *British Journal of Haematology*, **95**, 2–9.

Banavali, S., Silvestri, F., Hulette, B., *et al.* (1991). Expression of hematopoietic progenitor cell associated antigen CD34 in chronic myeloid leukemia. *Leukemia Research*, **15**, 603–8.

Barnes, D. J. & Melo, J. V. (2002). Cytogenetic and molecular genetic aspects of chronic myeloid leukemia. *Acta Haematologica*, **108**, 180–202.

Barosi, G., Ambrosetti, A., Finelli, C., *et al.* (1999). The Italian consensus conference on diagnostic criteria for myelofibrosis with myeloid metaplasia. *British Journal of Haematology*, **104**, 730–7.

Berkowicz, M., Rosner, E., Rechavi, G., *et al.* (1991). Atypical chronic myelomonocytic leukemia with eosinophilia and translocation (5;12): a new association. *Cancer Genetics and Cytogenetics*, **51**, 277–8.

Besses, C., Cervantes, F., Pereira, A., *et al.* (1999). Major vascular complications in essential thrombocythemia: a study of the predictive factors in a series of 148 patients. *Leukemia*, **13**, 150–4.

Buckley, M. G., McEuen, A. R., & Walls, A. F. (1999). The detection of mast cell subpopulations in formalin-fixed human tissues using a new monoclonal antibody specific for chymase. *Journal of Pathology*, **189**, 138–43.

Cervantes, F., Villamor, N., Esteve, J., *et al.* (1998). "Lymphoid" blast crisis of chronic myeloid leukaemia is associated with distinct clinicohaematological features. *British Journal of Haematology*, **100**, 123–8.

Cools, J., DeAngelo, D. J., Gotlib, J., *et al.* (2003). A tyrosine kinase created by fusion of the PDGFRA and FIP1L1 genes as a therapeutic target of imatinib in idiopathic hypereosinophilic syndrome. *New England Journal of Medicine*, **348**, 1201–14.

Dewald, G. W. & Wright, P. I. (1995). Chromosome abnormalities in the myeloproliferative disorders. *Seminars in Oncology*, **22**, 341–54.

Dupriez, B., Morel, P., Demory, J. L., *et al.* (1996). Prognostic factors in agnogenic myeloid metaplasia: a report of 195 cases with a new scoring system. *Blood*, **88**, 1013–8.

Escribano, L., Orfao, A., Villarrubia, J., *et al.* (1997). Sequential immunophenotypic analysis of mast cells in a case of systemic mast cell disease evolving to a mast cell leukemia. *Cytometry*, **30**, 98–102.

Facchetti, F., Tironi, A., Marocolo, D., *et al.* (1997). Histopathological changes in bone marrow biopsies from patients with chronic myeloid leukaemia after treatment with recombinant alpha-interferon. *Histopathology*, **31**, 3–11.

Gale, R. E. (2003). Pathogenic markers in essential thrombocythemia. *Current Hematology Reports*, **2**, 242–7.

George, T. I. & Arber, D. A. (2003). Pathology of the myeloproliferative diseases. *Hematology/Oncology Clinics of North America*, **17**, 1101–27.

Guyotat, D., Campos, L., Thomas, X., *et al.* (1990). Myelodysplastic syndromes: a study of surface markers and in vitro growth patterns. *American Journal of Hematology*, **34**, 26–31.

Hamazaki, M. & Mugishima, H. (1981). Agnogenic myelofibrosis in children: a case report and review of the literature. *Acta Pathologica Japonica*, **31**, 143–52.

Harris, N. L., Jaffe, E. S., Diebold, J., *et al.* (1999). The World Health Organization classification of neoplastic diseases of the hematopoietic and lymphoid tissues: report of the Clinical Advisory Committee meeting, Airlie House, Virginia, November, 1997. *Annals of Oncology*, **10**, 1419–32.

Harrison, C. N., Gale, R. E., Machin, S. J., & Linch, D. C. (1999). A large proportion of patients with a diagnosis of essential thrombocythemia do not have a clonal disorder and may be at lower risk of thrombotic complications. *Blood*, **93**, 417–24.

Horny, H. P., Ruck, P., Krober, S., & Kaiserling, E. (1997). Systemic mast cell disease (mastocytosis): general aspects and histopathological diagnosis. *Histology and Histopathology*, **12**, 1081–9.

Horny, H. P., Sillaber, C., Menke, D., *et al.* (1998). Diagnostic value of immunostaining for tryptase in patients with mastocytosis. *American Journal of Surgical Pathology*, **22**, 1132–40.

Horny, H. P., Sotlar, K., Sperr, W. R., & Valent, P. (2004). Systemic mastocytosis with associated clonal haematological non mast cell lineage disease: a histopathological challenge. *Journal of Clinical Pathology*, **57**, 604–8.

Huang, T. Y., Yam, L. T., & Li, C. Y. (1987). Radiological features of systemic mast-cell disease. *British Journal of Radiology*, **60**, 765–70.

Jaffe, E. S., Harris, N. L., Stein, H., & Vardiman, J. W., eds. (2001). *World Health Organization Classification of Tumours: Pathol-*

ogy and Genetics of Tumours of Haematopoietic and Lymphoid Tissues. Lyon: IARC Press.

Khalidi, H. S., Brynes, R. K., Medeiros, L. J., *et al.* (1998). The immunophenotype of blast transformation of chronic myelogenous leukemia: a high frequency of mixed lineage phenotype in "lymphoid" blasts and a comparison of morphologic, immunophenotypic, and molecular findings. *Modern Pathology*, **11**, 1211–21.

LeBrun, D. P., Pinkerton, P. H., Sheridan, B. L., Chen-Lai, J., Dube, I. D., & Poldre, P. A. (1991). Essential thrombocythemia with the Philadelphia chromosome and BCR-ABL gene rearrangement: an entity distinct from chronic myeloid leukemia and Philadelphia chromosome-negative essential thrombocythemia. *Cancer Genetics and Cytogenetics*, **54**, 21–5.

Li, W. V., Kapadia, S. B., Sonmez-Alpan, E., & Swerdlow, S. H. (1996). Immunohistochemical characterization of mast cell disease in paraffin sections using tryptase, CD68, myeloperoxidase, lysozyme, and CD20 antibodies. *Modern Pathology*, **9**, 982–8.

Macdonald, D., Aguiar, R. C., Mason, P. J., Goldman, J. M., & Cross, N. C. (1995). A new myeloproliferative disorder associated with chromosomal translocations involving 8p11: a review. *Leukemia*, **9**, 1628–30.

Manoharan, A. (1998). Idiopathic myelofibrosis: a clinical review. *International Journal of Hematology*, **68**, 355–62.

Melo, J. V. (1996). The molecular biology of chronic myeloid leukaemia. *Leukemia*, **10**, 751–6.

Mesa, R. A., Silverstein, M. N., Jacobsen, S. J., Wollan, P. C., & Tefferi, A. (1999). Population-based incidence and survival figures in essential thrombocythemia and agnogenic myeloid metaplasia: an Olmsted county study. *American Journal of Hematology*, **61**, 10–15.

Mesa, R. A., Hanson, C. A., Rajkumar, S. V., Schroeder, G., & Tefferi, A. (2000). Evaluation and clinical correlations of bone marrow angiogenesis in myelofibrosis with myeloid metaplasia. *Blood*, **15**, 3374–80.

Mesa, R. A., Hanson, C. A., Li, C. Y., *et al.* (2002). Diagnostic and prognostic value of bone marrow angiogenesis and megakaryocyte c-Mpl expression in essential thrombocythemia. *Blood*, **99**, 4131–7.

Murphy, S. (1999). Diagnostic criteria and prognosis in polycythemia vera and essential thrombocythemia. *Seminars in Hematology*, **36**, 9–13.

Murphy, S., Peterson, P., Iland, H., & Laszlo J. (1997). Experience of the Polycythemia Vera Study Group with essential thrombocythemia: a final report on diagnostic criteria, survival, and leukemic transition by treatment. *Seminars in Hematology*, **34**, 29–39.

Nand, S., Stock, W., Godwin, J., & Fisher, S. G. (1996). Leukemogenic risk of hydroxyurea therapy in polycythemia vera, essential thrombocythemia, and myeloid metaplasia with myelofibrosis. *American Journal of Hematology*, **52**, 42–6.

Orazi, A. (1995). CD34 immunoperoxidase staining for the diagnosis of myelodysplastic syndromes and chronic myeloid leukaemia. *Journal of Clinical Pathology*, **48**, 884.

Orazi, A., Cattoretti, G., & Sozzi, G. (1989). A case of chronic neutrophilic leukemia with trisomy 8. *Acta Haematologica*, **81**, 148–51.

Orazi, A., Neiman, R. S., Cualing, H., Heerema, N. A., & John, K. (1994). CD34 immunostaining of bone marrow biopsy specimens is a reliable way to classify the phases of chronic myeloid leukemia. *American Journal of Clinical Pathology*, **101**, 426–8.

Orazi, A., Shendrik, I., Servida, P., & Ponzoni, M. (2001). Angiogenesis in agnogenic myeloid metaplasia. *Modern Pathology*, **14**, 175A.

Pahl, H. L. (2003). PRV-1 mRNA expression and other molecular markers in polycythemia rubra vera. *Current Hematology Reports*, **2**, 231–6.

Pane, F., Frigeri, F., Sindona, M., *et al.* (1996). Neutrophilic-chronic myeloid leukemia: a distinct disease with a specific molecular marker (BCR/ABL with C3/A2 junction). *Blood*, **88**, 2410–4.

Pardanani, A. D., Morice, W. G., Hoyer, J. D., & Tefferi, A. (2003a). Chronic basophilic leukemia: a distinct clinicopathologic entity. *European Journal of Haematology*, **71**, 18–22.

Pardanani, A. D., Reeder, T. L., Kimlinger, T. K., *et al.* (2003b). Flt-3 and c-kit mutation studies in a spectrum of chronic myeloid disorders including systemic mast cell disease. *Leukemia Research*, **27**, 739–42.

Pardanani, A. D., Kimlinger, T., Reeder, T., Li, C. Y., & Tefferi, A. (2004). Bone marrow mast cell immunophenotyping in adults with mast cell disease: a prospective study of 33 patients. *Leukemia Research*, **28**, 777–83.

Pearson, T. C. (2001). Evaluation of diagnostic criteria in polycythemia vera. *Seminars in Hematology*, **38** (1 Suppl. 2), 21–4.

Prchal, J. T. (2001). Pathogenetic mechanisms of polycythemia vera and congenital polycythemic disorders. *Seminars in Hematology*, **38** (1 Suppl. 2), 10–20.

Reilly, J. T., Snowden, J. A., Spearing, R. L., *et al.* (1997). Cytogenetic abnormalities and their prognostic significance in idiopathic myelofibrosis: a study of 106 cases. *British Journal of Haematology*, **98**, 96–102.

Reiter, A., Sohal, J., Kulkarni, S., *et al.* (1998). Consistent fusion of ZNF198 to the fibroblast growth factor receptor-1 in the (58;13)(p11;q12) myeloproliferative syndrome. *Blood*, **92**, 1735–42.

Sekhar, M., Prentice, H. G., Popat, U., *et al.* (1996). Idiopathic myelofibrosis in children. *British Journal of Haematology*, **93**, 394–7.

Smith, J. D. & Lazarchick, J. (1999). Systemic mast cell disease with marrow and splenic involvement associated with chronic myelomonocytic leukemia. *Leukemia and Lymphoma* **32**, 391–4.

Tanzer, J. (1994). Clonality and karyotype studies in polycythemia vera. *Nouvelle Revue Française d' Hématologie*, **36**, 167–72.

Thiele, J. & Kvasnicka, H.-M. (2000). Thrombocytosis versus thrombocythemia: differential diagnosis of elevated platelet count. *Pathologe*, **21**, 31–8.

Thiele, J. & Kvasnicka, H.-M. (2005). Diagnostic impact of bone marrow histopathology in polycythemia vera (PV). *Histology and Histopathology*, **20**, 317–28.

Thiele, J., Kvasnicka, H.-M., Werden, C., Zankovich, R., Diehl, V., & Fischer, R. (1996). Idiopathic primary osteo-myelofibrosis: a clinico-pathological study on 208 patients with special emphasis on evolution, differentiation from essential thrombocythemia and variables of prognostic impact. *Leukemia and Lymphoma*, **22**, 303–17.

Thiele, J., Kvasnicka, H.-M., Boeltken, B., Zankovich, R., Diehl, V., & Fischer, R. (1999). Initial (prefibrotic) stages of idiopathic (primary) myelofibrosis (IMF): a clinicopathological study. *Leukemia*, **13**, 1741–8.

Thiele, J., Kvasnicka, H. M., Zankovich, R., & Diehl, V. (2000). Relevance of bone marrow features in the differential diagnosis between essential thrombocythemia and early stage idiopathic myelofibrosis. *Haematologica*, **85**, 1126–34.

Thiele, J., Kvasnicka, H. M., Facchetti, F., Franco, V., von Der Walt, J., & Orazi, A. (2005). European consensus on grading bone marrow fibrosis and assessment of cellularity. *Haematologica*, **90**, 1128–32.

Wang, J. K., Lin, D. T., Hsieh, H. C., Chuu, W. M., Wang, C. H., & Lin, K. S. (1990). Primary myelofibrosis in children: report of 4 cases. *Journal of the Formosan Medical Association*, **89**, 719–23.

Wolf, B. C., Banks, P. M., Mann, R. B., & Neiman, R. S. (1988). Splenic hematopoiesis in polycythemia vera: a morphologic and immunohistologic study. *American Journal of Clinical Pathology*, **89**, 69–75.

Yang, F., Tran, T.-A., Carlson, J. A., His, E. D., Ross, C. W., & Arber, D. A. (2000). Paraffin section immunophenotype of cutaneous and extracutaneous mast cell disease: comparison to other hematopoietic neoplasms. *American Journal of Surgical Pathology*, **24**, 703–9.

10

Myelodysplastic/myeloproliferative disorders

Introduction

The category of myelodysplastic/myeloproliferative disorders (MDS/MPD) includes malignant hematopoietic proliferations which, at the time of their initial presentation, display features of both myelodysplastic syndromes and myeloproliferative disorders (Oscier, 1997; Jaffe *et al.*, 2001). Cytopenias and dysplastic changes of any cell line may be seen, similar to the myelodysplastic syndromes. Elevated white blood cell counts, hypercellular marrows with fibrosis, and organomegaly, features more commonly associated with myeloproliferative disorders, may also be present. The presence of fibrosis alone in cases that are otherwise typical of myelodysplasia should not be placed in this category. The three best-defined mixed myeloproliferative and myelodysplastic syndromes are atypical chronic myeloid leukemia (atypical CML), chronic myelomonocytic leukemia (CMML), and juvenile myelomonocytic leukemia (JMML). Features that help in differentiating the chronic phase of CML from atypical CML and CMML are listed in Table 10.1.

Atypical chronic myeloid leukemia

Atypical CML (Bennett *et al.*, 1994) is a Philadelphia chromosome-negative and *BCR/ABL*-negative proliferative disorder that affects elderly patients, with an apparent male predominance. Its incidence is <2 cases for every 100 cases of t(9;22), *BCR/ABL*-positive CML (Jaffe *et al.*, 2001). Patients have some features of CML including splenomegaly, an elevated white blood cell count of predominantly granulocytic cells, and moderate anemia. The major characteristic which distinguishes atypical CML is dysgranulopoiesis, which is often severe. Moreover,

atypical CML may have an initial presentation more typical of myelodysplasia with a low white blood cell count and normal to decreased platelet counts (Oscier, 1996). The white blood cells are shifted to the left with immature granulocytes, including blast cells, promyelocytes, and myelocytes, representing 10% to 20% of peripheral blood white cells. Dysplastic neutrophils are typically seen (Fig. 10.1). Granulocytes may show typical pseudo-Pelger–Huët changes, "mononuclear" cell-like morphology due to nuclear condensation, and cytoplasmic hypogranularity. Monocytes are usually less than 10% of peripheral blood cells. In contrast to CML, basophilia is not prominent, usually accounting for less than 2% of peripheral blood white cells.

The bone marrow is hypercellular, with an elevated myeloid-to-erythroid ratio, and marrow fibrosis may be present (Fig. 10.2). The bone marrow biopsy demonstrates granulocytic hyperplasia with an increased proportion of blasts (<20%). These cells can be highlighted by immunostaining with CD34. Dysmegakaryopoiesis is easily identified. A predominance of small megakaryocytic forms, which can be similar in appearance to those seen in MDS, may be observed. The myeloid-to-erythroid ratio is usually less than 10 : 1, and there is no evidence of the Philadelphia chromosome by either routine karyotype or molecular studies for the *BCR/ABL* fusion product. Although some abnormalities of granulocyte nuclear lobation may be seen in CML, particularly in accelerated phase, atypical CML commonly has more typical dysplastic changes that may involve all cell lines (trilineage dysplasia). In addition to dysgranulopoiesis, dyserythropoiesis and megakaryocyte dysplasia are common, and megakaryocytes may be reduced in number with associated thrombocytopenia. Atypical CML is a more aggressive disease than CML, and progression usually occurs within two years

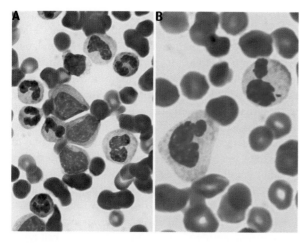

Figure 10.1. Atypical chronic myeloid leukemia (aCML). (A) Peripheral blood smear showing neutrophilia characterized by the presence of immature granulocytic cells. (B) Dysgranulopoiesis is a feature constantly seen in aCML. Note the abnormal chromatin clumping of the neutrophils.

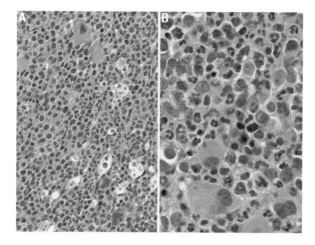

Figure 10.2. aCML. (A) Core biopsy showing a hypercellular bone marrow with increased granulopoiesis characterized by the presence of immature forms, including blasts, numerous neutrophils, and pleomorphic-appearing megakaryocytes. (B) High magnification showing a different case with hypolobated megakaryocytes and increased numbers of eosinophils, neutrophils, and blasts.

(Martiat *et al.*, 1991; Oscier, 1996). Patients may develop acute leukemia or may have bone marrow failure secondary to marked fibrosis.

Cytogenetic and molecular genetic studies are essential in the diagnosis of atypical CML to exclude t(9;22) or the *BCR/ABL* fusion product of usual-type CML. There is

Table 10.1. Features in the differential diagnosis of chronic phase of CML, atypical CML, and CMML.

Feature	CML	Atypical CML	CMML
Philadelphia chromosome/*BCR/ABL*	+	−	−
Peripheral blood white cell count	+++	++	+
Peripheral blood basophils	≥2%	<2%	<2%
Peripheral blood monocytes	<3%	3%–10%	Usually > 10%
Peripheral blood promyelocytes, myelocytes, and metamyelocytes	>20%	10%–20%	≥10%
Peripheral blood blasts	<2%	>2%	<2%
Granulocyte dysplasia	−	++	+
Bone marrow erythroid hyperplasia	−	−	+

no known defining cytogenetic abnormality for atypical CML, but del(20q11) and trisomy 8 have been reported (Jaffe *et al.*, 2001). Other ancillary studies, particularly immunophenotyping studies, do not usually help unless blast cell numbers are elevated.

Chronic myelomonocytic leukemia

CMML has features of both a myeloproliferative and a myelodysplastic syndrome. The disease has been divided into myelodysplastic and myeloproliferative subtypes on the basis of a white blood cell count of 13×10^9/L or higher for the myeloproliferative type and less than that number for the myelodysplastic type. Patients with leukocytosis of $>13 \times 10^9$/L have a higher incidence of splenomegaly (Bennett *et al.*, 1994). However, both subtypes show a similar degree of dysplastic changes. Since the percentage of bone marrow (or peripheral blood) blasts is the most important determinant of survival in CMML patients, the use of a white blood cell cutoff to separate the subtypes is probably arbitrary and of controversial prognostic value (Germing *et al.*, 1998).

The diagnosis requires a persistent peripheral blood monocytosis of more than 1×10^9/L, with a percentage of monocytes greater than 10% of the WBCs. The monocytes may be abnormal in appearance with bizarre nuclei and even cytoplasmic granules (Fig. 10.3). Promonocytes, with more immature nuclear chromatin, may be present in the blood, but monoblasts are usually not present or represent less than 2% of peripheral blood cells. If blasts and promonocytes account for 20% or more of the WBC, the diagnosis should be acute myeloid leukemia rather than

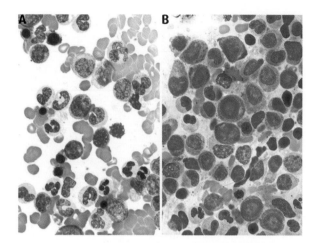

Figure 10.3. (A) Peripheral blood smear in a case of chronic myelomonocytic leukemia (CMML). Note the presence of monocytosis that includes both mature and immature forms. In addition, there are numerous granulocytes, with some showing nuclear hypolobation and hypogranularity. (B) Aspirate smear in CMML. Note how the monocytic forms are difficult to identify within a granulocyte-rich marrow cellularity. Esterase staining may be of benefit in confirming the presence of monocytic forms.

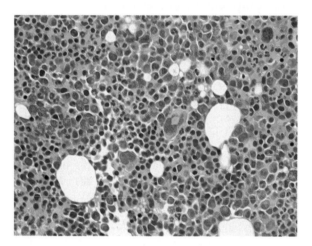

Figure 10.4. Core biopsy, chronic myelomonocytic leukemia (CMML-1). Increased M : E ratio and presence of dysplastic megakaryocytes.

CMML. The peripheral blood may demonstrate dysplastic changes typical of the myelodysplastic syndromes, or dysplastic changes may be minimal. Other changes in the peripheral blood are variable; however, mild anemia is usually seen. Although an elevated peripheral blood monocyte count is necessary for the diagnosis of CMML, such a diagnosis should never be made without examination of

the bone marrow. Some AMLs with monocytic blasts may show peripheral blood changes similar to those of CMML because of cytologic maturation of the blast cell population in the peripheral blood. The bone marrow of CMML is usually hypercellular and may demonstrate monocytic or granulocytic hyperplasia (Figs. 10.3, 10.4). When granulocytic hyperplasia is prominent, it may be difficult to distinguish the abnormal monocyte population from myelocytes. Nonspecific esterase cytochemical studies may be helpful in this setting, by highlighting the abnormal monocytes. Flow cytometry and immunohistochemistry may be useful in confirming the presence of myelomonocytic immunophenotypic markers including CD14, CD163, CD68, and CD64. Erythroid precursors and megakaryocytes may demonstrate prominent dysplastic changes, but these cell types are often normal in appearance. Ringed sideroblasts are present in increased numbers in some cases. Blast cell and promonocyte counts may be elevated up to 20%, and an elevation in blast cell numbers is associated with a poorer prognosis (Fenaux *et al.*, 1988; Storniolo *et al.*, 1990). When bone marrow blast and promonocyte counts are more than 20%, cases have previously been considered CMML in transformation, but are now diagnosed as AML.

The WHO classification scheme subdivides CMML into two subcategories, depending on the number of blasts found in the peripheral blood and bone marrow. These are CMML-1, with blasts <5% in the blood or <10% in the bone marrow, and CMML-2, which is characterized by blasts 5–19% in the blood or 10–19% in the bone marrow, or when Auer rods are present and the blast count is less than 20% in blood or marrow. A finding of >20% blasts in the blood or the bone marrow indicates AML rather than CMML.

Ancillary studies help in the differential diagnosis of CMML. Cytochemistry for non-specific esterase on the peripheral blood and bone marrow confirms the presence of an increase in monocytes and can help differentiate abnormal monocytes of CMML from myelocytes in CML and atypical CML. Flow cytometry and immunohistochemistry may be useful in confirming the presence of cells with monocytic differentiation. Cytogenetic and molecular genetic studies, particularly the absence of the Philadelphia chromosome and *BCR/ABL*, help in excluding CML. An additional subset, CMML with eosinophilia, may be diagnosed when the criteria for CMML are present, but in addition the eosinophil count in the peripheral blood is >1.5 × 10⁹/L. Patients in this category may have symptoms related to the degranulation of the eosinophils, comparable to those seen in hypereosinophilic syndrome (see Chapter 9). This subset should be designated as CMML-1 or CMML-2 with eosinophilia according to the above guidelines (Fig. 10.5). A proportion of these cases are associated

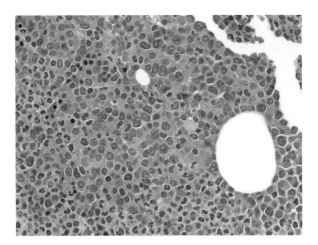

Figure 10.5. Chronic myelomonocytic leukemia (CMML-2) with eosinophilia. Increased numbers of immature myeloid elements, blasts included, and eosinophils are present.

with a t(5;12)(q33;p13) chromosome abnormality involving the *PDGFRβ* and *TEL* genes (Golub *et al.*, 1994; Steer & Cross, 2002). The resulting tyrosine kinase fusion protein activates the *RAS* signal transduction pathway. Mutations of *RAS* are detected in approximately one-third of CMML cases. Although detection of *RAS* mutations is not generally useful for diagnosis, abnormalities involving the *RAS* pathway are thought to be an important mechanism for this and other chronic myeloproliferative disorders, including CML.

The differential diagnosis between atypical CML and CMML may be difficult, but it is critical because of the worse prognosis of patients with atypical CML compared with CMML. CMML may be distinguished from atypical CML by peripheral blood features (Bennett *et al.*, 1994), but some overlap with atypical CML may occur (Table 10.1). Monocyte counts are slightly elevated in atypical CML but do not usually exceed 10%, whereas monocyte counts in CMML are usually above 10%. The degree of granulocyte dysplasia in CMML is also not as pronounced as is usually seen in atypical CML. Atypical CML demonstrates an increase in immature granulocytic cells, including blast cells, promyelocytes, and myelocytes, of up to 20% in the peripheral blood; these cell types are almost always below 10% in the blood of patients with CMML.

Juvenile myelomonocytic leukemia

JMML, a member of the WHO myelodysplastic/myeloproliferative diseases group, is described with the pediatric myelodysplastic syndromes in Chapter 7.

Other myelodysplastic/myeloproliferative syndromes

Some cases demonstrate features of both myelodysplasia and myeloproliferative syndromes and do not fit well into any of the previously mentioned categories. Many of these cases have typical features of myelodysplasia as well as an atypical finding more suggestive of a myeloproliferative disorder, such as marked marrow fibrosis, leukocytosis, or organomegaly. Such cases may be termed mixed myeloproliferative/myelodysplastic syndromes, not further classifiable, with a comment describing the atypical findings. One such syndrome has features of refractory anemia with ringed sideroblasts and thrombocythemia (acquired sideroblastic anemia associated with thrombocytosis). These cases have no sex predilection or specific cytogenetic abnormality and must be differentiated from the 5q− syndrome myelodysplasias. A mixed myeloproliferative–myelodysplastic disorder associated with isochromosome 17q has been described; it occurs with a male predominance in adults and is associated with severe hyposegmentation of neutrophil nuclei, monocytosis, and a high rate of transformation to AML. A poorly characterized myelodysplastic/myeloproliferative disease may also occur with mast cell disease.

REFERENCES

Bennett, J. M., Catovsky, D., Daniel, M. T., *et al.* (1994). The chronic myeloid leukemias: guidelines for distinguishing chronic granulocytic, atypical chronic myeloid, and chronic myelomonocytic leukemia. Proposals by the French–American–British Cooperative Leukemia group. *British Journal of Haematology*, **87**, 746–54.

Fenaux, P., Beuscart, R., Lai, J. L., Jouet, J. P., & Bauters, F. (1988). Prognostic factors in adult chronic myelomonocytic leukemia: an analysis of 107 cases. *Journal of Clinical Oncology*, **6**, 1417–24.

Germing, U., Gattermann, N., Minning, H., Heyll, A., & Aul, C. (1998). Problems in the classification of CMML: dysplastic versus proliferative type. *Leukemia Research*, **22**, 871–8.

Golub, T. R., Barker, G. F., Lovett, M., & Gilliland, D. G. (1994). Fusion of PDGF receptor to a novel *ets*-like gene, *tel*, in chronic myelomonocytic leukemia with t(5;12) chromosomal translocation. *Cell*, **77**, 307–16.

Jaffe, E. S., Harris, N. L., Stein, H., & Vardiman, J. W., eds. (2001). *World Health Organization Classification of Tumours: Pathology and Genetics of Tumours of Haematopoietic and Lymphoid Tissues*. Lyon: IARC Press.

Martiat, P., Michaux, J. L., & Rodhain, J. (1991). Philadelphia-negative (Ph−) chronic myeloid leukemia (CML): comparison with Ph+ CML and chronic myelomonocytic leukemia. *Blood*, **78**, 205–11.

Oscier, D. (1997). Atypical chronic myeloid leukemias. *Pathologie Biologie (Paris)*, **45**, 587–93.

Oscier, D. G. (1996). Atypical chronic myeloid leukemia, a distinct clinical entity related to the myelodysplastic syndrome? *British Journal of Haematology*, **92**, 582–6.

Steer, E. J. & Cross, N. C. (2002). Myeloproliferative disorders with translocations of chromosome 5q31-35: role of the platelet-derived growth factor receptor beta. *Acta Haematologica*, **107**, 113–22.

Storniolo, A. M., Moloney, W. C., Rosenthal, D. S., Cox, C., & Bennett, J. M. (1990). Chronic myelomonocytic leukemia. *Leukemia*, **4**, 766–70.

11

Chronic lymphoproliferative disorders and malignant lymphoma

Introduction

Lymphoproliferative disorders frequently involve the peripheral blood and bone marrow, and bone marrow studies may be performed for primary diagnosis or as a staging procedure in patients with lymphoproliferative disorders. A primary diagnosis with accurate classification can often be made on bone marrow samples alone, if a combined morphologic and immunophenotypic approach is used. The addition of molecular or cytogenetic studies can resolve some of the low percentage of cases that are equivocal after morphologic and immunophenotypic analysis.

Many of the low-grade B-cell lymphomas will involve the bone marrow, but the precise morphologic classification of these diseases is complicated by the fact that characteristic architectural patterns seen in lymph nodes involved by these diseases are not present in the bone marrow. Despite this, many of the low-grade B-cell lymphomas have characteristic immunophenotypes that allow for proper classification. Flow cytometric immunophenotyping of involved peripheral blood or bone marrow aspirate material allows for evaluation of the largest number of antigens, as well as confirming aberrant co-expression of antigens that are characteristic of certain disease types. However, paraffin section immunophenotyping, which can be performed on core or clot biopsy material, can also be used successfully to detect many antigens of interest in these cases. The characteristic immunophenotypic features of the various small B-cell lymphoid proliferations are summarized in Table 11.1.

Molecular genetic or cytogenetic studies may also be useful in selected cases to confirm the presence of a clonal population, when the differential diagnosis is between reactive and neoplastic lymphoid proliferations (Arber, 2000).

Clonality assays for immunoglobulin heavy chain, light chain or T-cell receptor gene rearrangements are most commonly performed either by Southern blot analysis or by polymerase chain reaction (PCR). Most bone marrow samples, however, do not have sufficient material available for Southern blot analysis, and PCR methods have become extremely valuable in the study of bone marrow material. Many gene rearrangement PCR studies may be performed on fresh or frozen aspirate material as well as decalcified, formalin-fixed biopsy material. These studies do not usually work well on samples that are mercuric chloride-fixed (e.g., B5 fixative).

In addition to antigen receptor gene rearrangement studies, evaluation for cytogenetic translocations specific to a disease type may be useful for classification of a lymphoproliferative disorder in the bone marrow (Arber, 2000). Fluorescence *in situ* hybridization studies (FISH) or PCR studies can be performed for the specific abnormality in question, or standard karyotype analysis may be useful in screening for a variety of translocations. Table 11.2 summarizes the various molecular abnormalities that most commonly occur in lymphoproliferative disorders, and their most common detection methods.

Small B-cell proliferations

The B-cell neoplasms that involve the bone marrow may be divided into small B-cell lymphoid neoplasms and aggressive B-cell lymphomas/leukemias. The small B-cell neoplasms often present with peripheral blood involvement and have many morphologic similarities, all showing a proliferation of predominantly small B lymphocytes. Therefore, immunophenotyping studies are essential for proper classification.

Table 11.1. Immunophenotypic findings of small B-cell lymphoid proliferations.

	CLL	B-PLL	MCL	FL	HCL	MZL
CD19	+	+	+	+	+	+
CD20	weak +/−	+	+	+	+	+
Immunoglobulin surface light chains	weak +/−	+	+	+	+	+
CD5	+	−/+	+	−	−	−
CD10	−	−	−	+	−/+	−
CD23	+	−/+	−	+/−	−	−
CD43	+	−/+	+	−	−	−[a]
CD103	−	−	−	−	+	−/+
DBA.44	−	−/+	−	−	+	+
FMC7	−	+	+	−/+	+	+
CYCLIN D1/BCL1	−	−	+	−	weak +/−	−
BCL2	+	+	+	+/−	+	+
BCL6	−	−	−	+	−	−

CLL, chronic lymphocytic leukemia; B-PLL, B-cell prolymphocytic leukemia, MCL, mantle cell lymphoma; FL, follicular lymphoma; HCL, hairy cell leukemia; MZL, marginal zone lymphoma.

+, positive; +/−, usually positive; −/+, usually negative; −, negative.

[a] up to 40% of non-splenic marginal zone cell lymphomas are CD43-positive.

Chronic lymphocytic leukemia/small lymphocytic lymphoma

Chronic lymphocytic leukemia (CLL) is a clonal proliferation of B cells that usually involves the bone marrow, peripheral blood, and lymph nodes. The term small lymphocytic lymphoma is usually reserved for the same disease with primarily lymph node involvement. CLL most commonly occurs in older adults, with a male predominance. The majority of cells are small lymphocytes with clumped nuclear chromatin and scant to moderately abundant cytoplasm, but this disease characteristically also shows admixed larger lymphocytes with moderately abundant cytoplasm and variably prominent nucleoli or a single distinct larger nucleolus, which are termed prolymphocytes (Fig. 11.1). The number of prolymphocytes is 10% or less in the peripheral blood of "usual" CLL (Bennett *et al.*, 1989). These larger cells often form aggregates in lymphoid tissues that are termed pseudofollicles or proliferation centers, but these aggregates are not always apparent on bone marrow biopsy material. A small proportion of paraimmunoblasts, cells that are larger and have a more prominent nucleolus than a prolymphocyte, are also seen

in the pseudofollicles or admixed with the small lymphocytes. The term CLL should be used for cases with 5000 or more peripheral blood lymphocytes, or 30% or more bone marrow involvement (Cheson *et al.*, 1996). Bone marrow examination is not required for the diagnosis of CLL, but immunophenotyping studies of an involved site, such as peripheral blood, are necessary to exclude one of the other disorders of small B cells.

Although both bone marrow aspirate and biopsy material are involved by CLL, the biopsy material is most useful for evaluating the degree and pattern of bone marrow involvement. CLL may infiltrate in a nodular, interstitial, diffuse, or mixed pattern, with nodular involvement having the best prognosis and diffuse having the worst (Pangalis *et al.*, 1984; Rozman *et al.*, 1984).

CLL may be associated with autoimmune disorders, including autoimmune hemolytic anemia, idiopathic thrombocytopenic purpura, red cell aplasia, and neutropenia (Diehl & Ketchum, 1998; Pritsch *et al.*, 1998). Therefore, the bone marrow should be evaluated for signs of these diseases, in addition to evaluation for involvement by the lymphoproliferative disorder.

To distinguish CLL from other lymphoproliferative disorders, immunophenotyping studies are essential to confirm the diagnosis. CLL is a clonal B-cell neoplasm, but surface CD20 and immunoglobulin light chains are characteristically weak and may not be detectable in some cases. However, the B cells show aberrant co-expression of the T-cell antigen CD5, as well as CD43, combined with CD23 expression. The combination of weak CD20 and light chain expression with CD5 and CD23 is characteristic of the disease (DiGiuseppe & Borowitz, 1998; Jaffe *et al.*, 2001). The cells also characteristically express CD19 and CD79a, lack CD10 and FMC7, and show weak to no expression of CD22 and CD79b. CD38 and ZAP-70 expression are detected in a subset of cases. These antigens are associated with unmutated immunoglobulin V_H genes and more aggressive disease (Damle *et al.*, 1999; Crespo *et al.*, 2003).

Molecular studies are usually not necessary for the diagnosis of CLL, although all cases undergo immunoglobulin heavy chain gene rearrangements. Characteristic cytogenetic abnormalities in CLL include deletions of 13q14, 11q22–23, 17p13, and 6q21, and trisomy 12, with 13q deletions having the best prognosis and 17p deletions the worst (Dohner *et al.*, 1999). Lack of mutation of immunoglobulin V_H genes has also been associated with more aggressive disease in CLL (Hamblin *et al.*, 1999; Stilgenbauer *et al.*, 2002).

Prolymphocytoid and large cell transformation (Richter syndrome) may occur in CLL (Fig. 11.2). Prolymphocytoid transformation occurs in patients with documented

Table 11.2. Most common molecular abnormalities and detection methods in chronic lymphoproliferative disorders.

Gene studied	Chromosomal site	Most common disease associations	Most common detection methods
Immunoglobulin heavy chain (IgH) rearrangements	14q32	B-cell neoplasms[a]	PCR, SB
Immunoglobulin kappa light chain (Igκ) rearrangements	2p11	B-cell neoplasms	SB, PCR
J_H/BCL-1	t(11;14)(q13;q32)	Mantle cell lymphoma	Cyclin D1 IHC, PCR, FISH, Karyotype
J_H/BCL-2	t(14;18)(q32;q21)	Follicular lymphoma, some diffuse large B-cell lymphomas	PCR, SB, FISH, Karyotype
API2/MLT	t(11;18)(q21;q21)	Extranodal marginal zone lymphoma	FISH, PCR
BCL-6 translocations	t(3;n)(q27;n)	Some diffuse large B-cell lymphomas	SB
C-MYC translocations	t(8;n)(q24;n)	Burkitt lymphoma	Karyotype, FISH
T-cell receptor β chain (TCRβ) rearrangements	7q34	T-cell neoplasms[a]	SB
T-cell receptor γ chain (TCRγ) rearrangements	7q15	T-cell neoplasms[a]	PCR
NPM/ALK	t(2;5)(p23;q35)	Anaplastic large cell lymphoma	ALK1 IHC, FISH, RT-PCR

PCR, polymerase chain reaction; SB, Southern blot analysis; IHC, immunohistochemistry; FISH, fluorescence *in situ* hybridization; RT-PCR, reverse transcriptase PCR.

[a] Lineage infidelity may occur in some neoplasms, particularly lymphoblastic leukemias and lymphomas, which may result in detection of aberrant gene rearrangements.

CLL that develop over 55% peripheral blood prolymphocytes. The polymphocytoid cells are often more heterogeneous than the prolymphocytes of "*de novo*" prolymphocytic leukemia. Large cell transformation requires the presence of confluent sheets of large cells, which may have either a typical large cell or immunoblast appearance. Another process related to transformation which may be seen in lymph nodes of patients with CLL is the so-called paraimmunoblastic transformation (Espinet, 2002). Cells with morphologic and immunophenotypic features of classical Hodgkin lymphoma may also be present admixed with typical CLL cells, and these cases may recur as classical Hodgkin lymphoma (Momose *et al.*, 1992).

B-cell prolymphocytic leukemia

The term B-cell prolymphocytic leukemia (B-PLL) is reserved for cases that present *de novo* with over 55% medium to large peripheral blood cells with a prominent, usually single, nucleolus. This disease involves the peripheral blood (usually with a markedly elevated white blood cell count), bone marrow, and spleen, most commonly in older males. The prolymphocytes usually diffusely involve the bone marrow and show prominent nucleoli on tissue sections (Fig. 11.3). The immunophenotype of

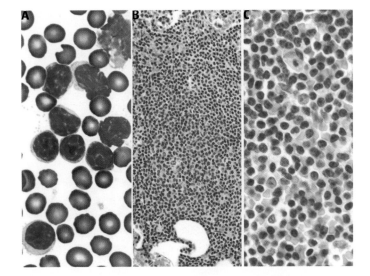

Figure 11.1. Chronic lymphocytic leukemia (CLL). (A) The peripheral blood shows an increase in small lymphocytes, most of which have clumped nuclear chromatin. Admixed smudged cells are commonly seen in the blood. (B) The bone marrow biopsy in this case shows a predominantly nodular pattern of infiltration that is away from the bony trabeculae. (C) Higher magnification shows mostly small round lymphocytes with admixed larger lymphocytes or prolymphocytes.

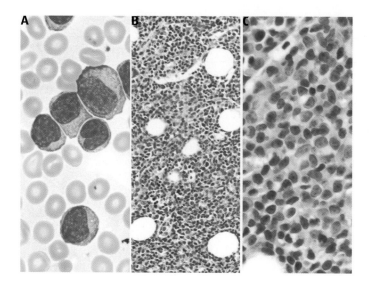

Figure 11.2. Prolymphocytic transformation of chronic lymphocytic leukemia. (A) This patient with a prior diagnosis of CLL now shows an increase in peripheral blood prolymphocytes, which are larger cells with abundant cytoplasm and a central prominent nucleolus. (B) The bone marrow shows an interstitial and diffuse infiltration. (C) On higher magnification, admixed intermediate-sized prolymphocytes with more open chromatin are easily identified.

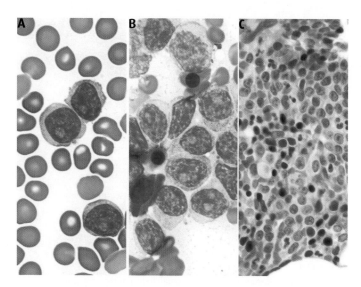

Figure 11.3. B-cell prolymphocytic leukemia (B-PLL). (A) The peripheral blood shows an elevated white blood cell count, with most of the lymphocytes showing abundant cytoplasm and a single prominent nucleolus. (B) The bone marrow aspirate shows a similar population of cells. (C) The bone marrow shows a nodular infiltrate with intermediate-sized prolymphocytes.

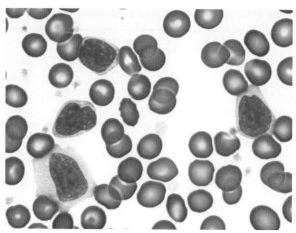

Figure 11.4. Atypical chronic lymphocytic leukemia (a-CLL). The peripheral blood shows scattered prolymphocytes as well as smaller lymphocytes, many of which have cleaved nuclei. Despite the atypical morphology, this proliferation showed a monotypic B-cell immunophenotype with expression of CD5 and CD23, typical of CLL.

B-PLL differs from CLL by usually showing bright CD20 and monotypic light chain expression, and expression of FMC7 in most cases. CD5 expression is only seen in approximately one-third of cases and CD23 is often not expressed in B-PLL.

All cases undergo immunoglobulin heavy chain gene rearrangements. Deletions of 11q23 and 13q14 may occur, and up to 20% of cases may have t(11;14)(q13;q32) (Brito-Babapulle *et al.*, 1987a; Lens *et al.*, 2000). The presence of this translocation raises the possibility that some cases of B-PLL may represent variants of mantle cell lymphoma. Other lymphoma types, including splenic marginal zone lymphoma, may also mimic B-PLL.

Atypical CLL and mixed CLL/PLL

Although not included in the recently published World Health Organization *Classification of Tumours of Haematopoietic and Lymphoid Tissues* (Jaffe *et al.*, 2001), categories of atypical CLL (a-CLL) and mixed CLL/PLL are used by many hematopathologists. Bone marrow involvement by other more well-characterized types of lymphoma should be excluded before such a diagnosis is made. Atypical CLL refers to cases with typical CLL morphology but an unusual immunophenotype, or to cases with the characteristic immunophenotype but unusual morphologic features (Fig. 11.4). Unusual immunophenotypic features of a-CLL include bright surface CD20 and immunoglobulin light chain expression or FMC7 expression. Unusual morphologic features include the presence of cleaved, notched, or irregular nuclear contours of small lymphocytes. Mixed CLL/PLL, or mixed cell-type CLL, are terms used for *de novo* cases that show 10–55% peripheral blood prolymphocytes. There is a great deal of overlap between cases described as a-CLL and mixed CLL/PLL, and both categories have an increased frequency of trisomy 12 and appear to have a more aggressive clinical course than typical cases of CLL.

Lymphoplasmacytic lymphoma

This lymphoma type is discussed in Chapter 12, with plasma cell disorders.

Hairy cell leukemia

Hairy cell leukemia (HCL) is a relatively uncommon clonal B-cell proliferation that occurs most frequently in elderly men (Pettitt *et al.*, 1999). Neoplastic cells most often are localized to the peripheral blood, bone marrow, and splenic red pulp, but peripheral blood involvement is usually at a low level. Patients usually present with pancytopenia, monocytopenia, splenomegaly, and no lymphadenopathy. Circulating tumor cells are small to medium size with oval to bean-shaped nuclei with homogeneous nuclear chromatin (Fig.11.5). The cells characteristically have abundant clear to slightly basophilic cytoplasm with cytoplasmic projections or "hairs," although these projections are a somewhat non-specific finding. Bone marrow aspirate smears from these patients are frequently aparticulate due to the extensive reticulin marrow fibrosis that is present. The marrow may be diffusely or partially infiltrated in an interstitial pattern by a uniform population of regularly spaced small lymphoid cells with moderately abundant clear cytoplasm (Fig. 11.5). These cells may be overlooked or mistaken for erythroid precursors on the biopsy material, particularly in cases with partial involvement.

Historically, hairy cell leukemia has been diagnosed by the demonstration of tartrate-resistant acid phosphatase (TRAP) by cytochemistry or ribosomal lamellar complexes by electron microscopy in the small lymphoid cells (Chang *et al.*, 1992). However, cytochemical staining is often difficult to interpret due to the small number of neoplastic cells in the peripheral blood or aparticulate aspirates of some patients, and most laboratories no longer offer routine electron microscopy. Immunophenotyping studies are useful to confirm the presence of a CD20-positive B-cell population in the marrow. If sufficient cells are available for flow cytometry studies, the B cells can be shown to have monotypic light chain expression with expression of FMC7,

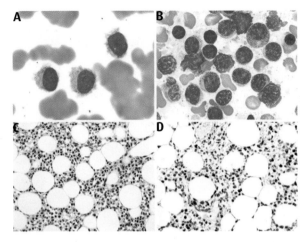

Figure 11.5. (A) Hairy cell leukemia (HCL) in the peripheral blood. The white blood cell count is often low, but the lymphocytes have homogeneous nuclear chromatin and cytoplasmic projections. Hairy cell leukemia in the bone marrow: (B) the bone marrow aspirate shows less obvious villous projections; (C) the bone marrow biopsy shows a subtle interstitial infiltrate on H&E sections. The infiltrate, however, stains for CD20 (shown) as well as DBA.44 and TRAP (D) by immunohistochemistry.

CD11c, CD25, and CD103 (Matutes *et al.*, 1994). Unlike CLL or mantle cell lymphoma, these B cells do not express CD5 or CD43. A subset of cases may express CD10. By immunohistochemistry, the hairy cells are usually positive for DBA.44, in contrast to most cases of chronic lymphocytic leukemia, but this marker is not specific for hairy cell leukemia (Salomon-Nguyen *et al.*, 1996). TRAP antibodies are also now available for immunohistochemistry and are useful in many cases (Hoyer *et al.*, 1997). In most cases, the detection of CD20-positive cells with the characteristic morphologic features, the pattern of bone marrow infiltration, and detection of combined DBA.44 and TRAP expression, in the absence of CD5 or CD43, are sufficient to make the diagnosis. Hairy cell leukemia is reported to show weak nuclear expression of cyclin D1 (Bosch *et al.*, 1995), a marker usually considered specific for mantle cell lymphoma; however, the other morphologic and immunophenotypic features of these cases would not suggest a diagnosis of mantle cell lymphoma. Although abnormalities of chromosome 5 are relatively common in hairy cell leukemia, no recurring cytogenetic abnormality is associated with this disease (Haglund *et al.*, 1994). Immunoglobulin heavy chain gene rearrangements, however, are present in all cases.

The term hairy cell leukemia variant has been used for cases of B-cell proliferations with cytoplasmic projections, similar to hairy cell leukemia, but prominent nucleoli more

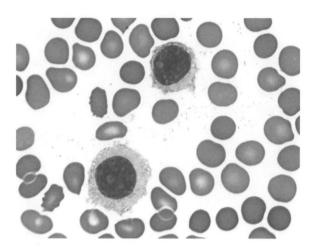

Figure 11.6. Hairy cell variant in the peripheral blood. The cells have villous cytoplasmic projections, similar to classical hairy cell leukemia, as well as a single prominent nucleolus, similar to prolymphocytes.

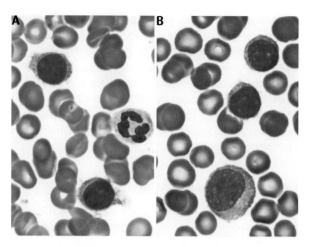

Figure 11.7. Splenic marginal zone lymphoma in the peripheral blood. The lymphocytes often show unipolar or bipolar cytoplasmic projections (A), but in many cases the peripheral blood lymphocytes do not show such obvious cytoplasmic changes (B).

typical of prolymphocytic leukemia (Catovsky *et al.*, 1984) (Fig. 11.6). The white blood cell count is usually elevated, in contrast to the leukopenia commonly seen in usual-type hairy cell leukemia. The immunophenotype may resemble that of typical HCL, but CD25 is usually negative (Matutes *et al.*, 2003). Some of these cases may represent peripheral blood involvement by other lymphomas, particularly splenic marginal zone lymphoma. It may not be possible to definitely distinguish hairy cell leukemia variant from splenic marginal zone lymphoma based on peripheral blood and bone marrow samples, but the pattern of splenic involvement differs for these diseases. The pattern of disease is predominantly red pulp in hairy cell leukemia and hairy cell leukemia variant, and predominantly white pulp in splenic marginal zone lymphoma.

Marginal zone lymphomas

There are at least three different types of marginal zone lymphoma: splenic, nodal, and extranodal. All of them may involve the peripheral blood and bone marrow, although peripheral blood involvement is more common in the splenic type, originally described as splenic lymphoma with circulating villous lymphocytes (SLVL) (Isaacson *et al.*, 1994). The peripheral blood cells are usually small to medium in size with moderately abundant cytoplasm (Fig. 11.7). Some cases will show unipolar or bipolar cytoplasmic projections that may mimic hairy cells. Some cells may show prominent nucleoli. In the bone marrow, splenic marginal zone lymphoma may have prominent intrasinusoidal infiltration (Franco *et al.*, 1996). Intrasinusoidal

infiltration, however, is not specific for splenic marginal zone lymphoma and can be observed in other types of lymphoma, particularly in cases associated with splenomegaly and peripheral blood lymphocytosis (Costes *et al.*, 2002).

Marginal zone lymphoma generally forms non-paratrabecular nodular aggregates composed of small lymphocytes with round to slightly irregular nuclei, but mixed patterns of infiltration may be present (Fig. 11.8). The lymphoid cells are monotypic B cells with CD20 expression and lack expression of CD5 or CD10. CD43 expression is not usually seen in cases of splenic marginal zone lymphoma, but may be present in 30–40% of the non-splenic types (Lai *et al.*, 1999).

Immunoglobulin heavy chain gene rearrangements are characteristically present in these diseases, and a subset of the extranodal marginal zone lymphomas, particularly those arising in the stomach and lung, demonstrate t(11;18) involving the *API2/MALT1* genes (Dierlamm *et al.*, 1999). Trisomy 3 is also common in these lymphomas (Dierlamm *et al.*, 1996). Other translocations that involve the immunoglobulin heavy chain gene on chromosome 14 occur in non-splenic extranodal marginal zone lymphomas and include the t(14;18) involving the *MALT1* gene (not the *BCL2* gene) (10%), the t(3;14) involving the *FOXP1* gene (10%), and the t(1;14)(q21–22;q32), involving the *BCL10* gene (<5%) (Streubel *et al.*, 2004).

Because some cases have abundant clear cytoplasm (monocytoid B cells), the differential diagnosis of marrow involvement by marginal zone lymphoma may include hairy cell leukemia. The pattern of bone marrow involvement by the two diseases, however, is different, with hairy cell leukemia showing patchy or diffuse interstitial involvement and marginal zone lymphoma forming focal non-paratrabecular lymphoid aggregates. Marginal zone lymphomas are also usually CD103- and TRAP-negative and may express CD43. The differential diagnosis with other chronic lymphoproliferative disorders may be more difficult. Although lack of CD5, CD23, or CD10 expression helps to rule out other types of small B-cell lymphoma this "triple negative" immunoprofile is not entirely specific for marginal zone lymphoma, since CD5-positive and rarely CD10-positive cases have been observed (Ferry *et al.*, 1996; Xu *et al.*, 2002). In addition, this immunophenotype does not entirely exclude the possibility of bone marrow involvement by CD10-negative follicular center cell lymphoma. Follicular lymphomas, however, usually show a paratrabecular pattern of marrow involvement.

Follicular lymphoma

Follicular lymphomas often involve the bone marrow and may also have significant involvement of the peripheral blood (Fig. 11.9). When the blood is involved, the lymphocytes may be variable in size, but usually show relatively scant cytoplasm. Although nuclear cleaves are a characteristic feature of this lymphoma type, they may be difficult to detect on blood smears. The bone marrow may be diffusely involved, but most commonly shows a paratrabecular pattern of infiltration (Lambertenghi-Deliliers *et al.*, 1992). The lymphoma cells show a mixture of small cleaved and large non-cleaved cells, and the paratrabecular aggregates are associated with focal reticulin fibrosis. Because of the fibrosis associated with the lymphoma infiltrate, aspirate smears may not demonstrate an obvious abnormality. Rare cases with diffuse involvement of the marrow will show the presence of neoplastic follicles, similar to the pattern of lymph node involvement (Torlakovic *et al.*, 2002). Most cases, however, do not show a follicular pattern in the marrow, but they may be graded based on the number of large cells in a fashion similar to that described in lymph nodes. The WHO criteria for grading are as follows: Grade 1, 0–5 large non-cleaved cells per high-power field (hpf); Grade 2, 6–15 large non-cleaved cells per hpf; Grade 3, more than 15 large non-cleaved cells per hpf (Jaffe *et al.*, 2001). Discordant grades, however, commonly occur between lymph node and bone marrow involvement (Robertson *et al.*, 1991).

Although immunophenotyping and molecular genetic studies may be useful in confirming a diagnosis of bone marrow involvement by follicular lymphoma, the morpho-

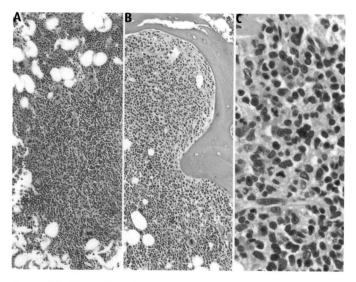

Figure 11.8. Marginal zone lymphoma of the bone marrow showing a nodular (A) and paratrabecular (B) pattern of involvement. Higher magnification (C) shows mostly small lymphocytes with irregular nuclear contours and smaller numbers of individual large cells.

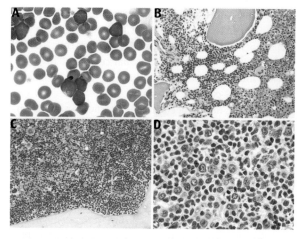

Figure 11.9. Follicular lymphoma. (A) In the peripheral blood, a subset of cells may have cleaved nuclei. The bone marrow infiltrate is usually paratrabecular, but may show a mixed pattern as seen in (B), with both paratrabecular and interstitial infiltrates. (C) This hypercellular marrow shows hyperplastic marrow as well as an extensive paratrabecular infiltrate. (D) The cells include a mix of small cleaved cells as well as variable numbers of large cells.

logic features are usually sufficient. Although a mixed paratrabecular and non-paratrabecular pattern of disease may be seen with mantle cell lymphoma, follicular lymphoma usually shows a more pure paratrabecular pattern and demonstrates a more heterogeneous cell population than mantle cell lymphoma. Reactive lymphoid aggregates do not normally occur in a paratrabecular location. The presence of definite lymphoid aggregates immediately adjacent to bone with fibrosis and no intervening fat should be considered highly suspicious for lymphoma in a patient with no prior history of disease, and diagnostic of involvement in patients with known follicular lymphoma.

Immunohistochemical studies may be misleading in evaluation of lymphoid aggregates of patients with follicular lymphoma, as this lymphoma type characteristically has numerous reactive T lymphocytes admixed with the lymphoma cells. Therefore, the detection of a mixed T and B cell population may incorrectly be interpreted as evidence of a reactive population. Such a population in a paratrabecular location should not be assumed to represent a reactive lymphoid aggregate. Detection of CD10 expression in the atypical lymphoid proliferation can be useful in detecting follicular lymphoma, but CD10 expression is often focally or completely lost in cases with marrow involvement, and the absence of this marker should not be used to rule out disease involvement. If sufficient lymphoma cells are aspirated, or if peripheral blood involvement is present, flow cytometry immunophenotyping may be useful. This lymphoma is CD20-positive, B lineage with monotypic light chain expression, and no CD5 or CD43 expression. As previously mentioned, detection of CD10 on the B cells is useful in classifying the process as follicular center cell in origin, but this immunophenotype may also be seen in a subset of diffuse large B-cell lymphomas.

Cytogenetic and molecular genetic studies may also be useful in classifying this disease type. Follicular lymphomas all undergo immunoglobulin heavy chain gene rearrangements, but somatic mutations of the gene are common and the rearrangement may not be detectable by polymerase chain reaction methods. However, most follicular lymphomas demonstrate t(14;18)(q32;q21) involving the immunoglobulin heavy chain gene on chromosome 14 and the *bcl-2* gene on chromosome 18. Karyotype, FISH, or PCR analysis may detect this translocation.

Mantle cell lymphoma

Mantle cell lymphoma (MCL) also frequently involves the peripheral blood and bone marrow (Wasman *et al.*, 1996; Cohen *et al.*, 1998) (Fig. 11.10). In the blood, the lymphoma cells may be round or irregular and may appear similar to peripheral blood involvement by follicular lymphoma. Although nucleoli are usually not prominent in mantle cell lymphoma, they may be seen in some cases in blood and marrow, suggesting prolymphocytic leukemia (Schlette

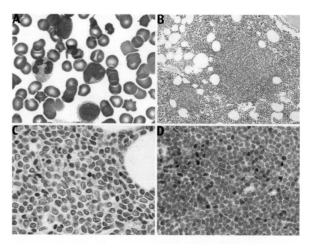

Figure 11.10. Mantle cell lymphoma (MCL) frequently involves the peripheral blood (A) and tends to show irregular cells, some of which may have prominent nucleoli. (B) The bone marrow in this case shows a nodular infiltrate, which on higher (C) power shows a monotonous population of small lymphocytes. (D) A subset of the infiltrate shows nuclear immunoreactivity with cyclin D1, a diagnostic feature of mantle cell lymphoma.

et al., 2001). The marrow may be diffusely involved, but a mixed paratrabecular and non-paratrabecular pattern is most common. Unlike follicular lymphoma, the lymphoid infiltrate is a homogeneous population of small cells that may have admixed epithelioid histiocytes.

The blastoid variant of mantle cell lymphoma shows finer nuclear chromatin and may be confused with lymphoblastic lymphoma. The cells of this type of mantle cell lymphoma, however, have the same immunophenotype as the other MCL cases and are TdT-negative, in contrast to lymphoblasts. Rare pleomorphic variants of blastoid MCL have also been reported (Ott *et al.*, 1998).

Immunophenotypic studies are useful in making the diagnosis of mantle cell lymphoma. By flow cytometry, the cells are monotypic B cells with bright CD20 and light chain expression, and aberrant CD5 expression. The cells also frequently mark with FMC7, but do not express CD23, helping to exclude chronic lymphocytic leukemia/small lymphocytic lymphoma. By immunohistochemistry, the B cells aberrantly express CD43 and show nuclear expression of cyclin D1. This immunophenotype is characteristic of mantle cell lymphoma.

Detection of immunoglobulin heavy chain gene rearrangements, even by PCR, is usually not difficult in this disease, and up to 90% of cases demonstrate t(11;14)(q13;q32) involving the immunoglobulin heavy chain gene and the *bcl-1/CCND1/PRAD1* gene of chromosome 18 (Arber, 2000). Detection of t(11;14) is best performed by FISH, as only

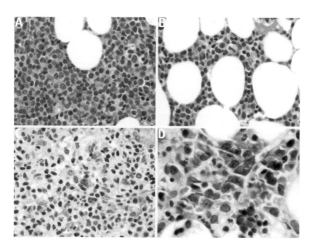

Figure 11.11. Large B-cell lymphoma. The bone marrow infiltration is usually diffuse (A), but an interstitial pattern may also occur (B). T-cell/histiocyte-rich large B-cell lymphoma (C) tends to form diffuse areas of infiltration. Most cells are small T lymphocytes with varying numbers of histiocytes and only rare atypical large cells (center), which immunoreact as B cells with CD20 or other B-lineage markers. (D) Intravascular large B-cell lymphoma. Clusters of large cells, which mark as B cells, are present within vascular channels.

approximately 40% of translocation involves the major translocation cluster that is detected by PCR methods. Quantitative PCR methods for cyclin D1 RNA expression will also detect the majority of cases.

Aggressive B-cell lymphomas

Diffuse large B-cell lymphoma

When diffuse large B-cell lymphoma involves the bone marrow, it is usually extensive and fairly easy to identify. The lymphoma cells most commonly show chromatin clearing and multiple small nucleoli (Fig. 11.11). Some cases display immunoblastic morphology, with over 90% of cells showing a central prominent nucleolus. These cells usually have more abundant, basophilic cytoplasm. Some cases with immunoblastic morphology will show plasmacytoid features, and without clinical correlation it may not be possible to distinguish these cases from anaplastic subtypes of multiple myeloma. Pleomorphic and anaplastic variants of diffuse large B-cell lymphoma may be confused with metastatic carcinoma. Demonstration of CD20 expression is sufficient for the diagnosis in most cases. A subset of cases, however, may show loss of CD20 expression *de novo* or after treatment with CD20-directed antibody therapies,

and additional B-lineage markers, such as CD79a, PAX5, or CD45RA, may be useful to confirm the cell lineage (Chu *et al.*, 2002). Although immunoglobulin heavy chain gene rearrangements are usually detectable in these cases, molecular studies are generally not necessary for diagnosis.

Discordance of morphology, such as bone marrow involvement by low-grade, small cleaved cell lymphoma, is relatively common in patients with nodal diffuse large cell lymphoma (Robertson *et al.*, 1991). Therefore, small lymphocyte proliferations in the bone marrow should be considered with suspicion in patients with a history of large cell lymphoma.

T-cell/histiocyte-rich large B-cell lymphoma

Although most large B-cell lymphomas in the bone marrow present with diffuse sheets of large neoplastic cells, a few exceptions exist. One is bone marrow involvement by T-cell/histiocyte-rich large B-cell lymphoma. This lymphoma shows a predominance of small T lymphocytes and histiocytes with less frequent admixed large neoplastic B cells (Fig. 11.11). Immunohistochemical studies are often necessary to confirm the presence of the neoplastic CD20-positive B-cell population. This lymphoma type may be easily confused with marrow involvement by nodular lymphocyte-predominant Hodgkin lymphoma, and distinguishing the two may not be possible on bone marrow material alone.

Intravascular large B-cell lymphoma

Bone marrow involvement by intravascular large B-cell lymphoma may also be subtle (Yegappan *et al.*, 2001). Patients with this type of lymphoma present with a variety of symptoms that may include skin lesions and neurologic symptoms. A diagnosis of lymphoma is often not suspected. The marrow may appear normal on low magnification, with only small clusters of large cells in vessels present on higher power (Fig. 11.11). These clusters are easily identified with a CD20 immunohistochemical stain.

Burkitt and Burkitt-like lymphoma

Burkitt and Burkitt-like lymphoma are morphologically, immunophenotypically, and genetically similar to L3 leukemia of the FAB classification of acute lymphoid leukemias (see Chapter 8) (Dayton *et al.*, 1994), but the term lymphoma is arbitrarily used when the marrow is less than 25% involved by the disease. When the marrow is involved, diffuse aggregates of lymphoma cells are present. In Burkitt lymphoma, the cells are medium-sized and uniform with moderately abundant, basophilic cytoplasm. On Wright–Giemsa-stained smears, cytoplasmic vacuoles are commonly seen. The lymphoma cells have uniformly sized round nuclei with fine nuclear chromatin and multiple small nucleoli. Mitotic figures are common and tingible body macrophages are often numerous. Burkitt-like lymphoma differs by less uniformity in cell size with more pleomorphism and more prominent, often single, nucleoli.

These tumors are CD20-positive, monotypic B-cell neoplasms, and usually express CD10, while negative for CD5, bcl-2, and TdT. In addition to their high mitotic rate, they show a near-100% proliferative rate with Ki-67 staining. Such staining is often helpful in the differential diagnosis of diffuse large B-cell lymphoma and Burkitt-like lymphoma. These tumors have immunoglobulin heavy chain gene rearrangements and translocations involving the *c-MYC* gene. The most common translocation is t(8;14)(q24;q32), involving the immunoglobulin heavy chain gene, but translocations involving the kappa or lambda light chain genes of 2q11 or 22q11, respectively, also occur. These translocations are best detected by karyotype analysis or FISH.

Lymphoblastic leukemia/lymphoma

Similar to Burkitt lymphoma/leukemia, lymphoblastic lymphoma and leukemia are arbitrarily distinguished by the degree of bone marrow involvement. Cases with less than 25% marrow involvement are usually considered as lymphoma. These diseases may be of precursor B or T lineage and usually diffusely infiltrate the marrow. They are discussed in more detail in Chapter 8.

T and NK/T-cell lymphoma

T-cell prolymphocytic leukemia

T-cell prolymphocytic leukemia (T-PLL) (Table 11.3) is a clonal proliferation that usually presents with a markedly elevated white blood cell count of 100×10^9/L or higher in elderly patients (Matutes *et al.*, 1991; Bartlett & Longo, 1999). A similar, but sometimes more indolent, disease occurs in younger patients with ataxia–telangiectasia (Taylor *et al.*, 1996; Garand *et al.*, 1998). The typical patient presents with organomegaly and lymphadenopathy, in addition to the marked lymphocytosis. Skin lesions, anemia, and thrombocytopenia are also common. Bone marrow involvement may be patchy and interstitial, diffuse, or a mixture of interstitial and diffuse, and reticulin fibrosis is common. Two different morphologic subtypes occur

Table 11.3. Immunophenotypic, molecular genetic, and viral association findings of small to medium-sized T- or NK-cell lymphoid neoplasms.

	T-PLL	T-LGL	NK NEOPLASMS	ATLL	MF/SS
CD2	+	+	+	+	+
sCD3	+	+	−	+	+
cCD3	+	+	+	+	+
CD4	+	−	−	+	+
CD5	+	+	−	+	+
CD7	+	+	+	−	−/+
CD8	−	+	−/+	−	−
CD25	−	−	−	+	−
CD56	−	+/−	+	−	−
CD57	−	+/−	+/−	−	−
TIA-1/ GRANZYME B	−	+	+	−	−
EBV	−	−	+	−	−
HTLV-1	−	−	−	+	−
TCR gene rearrangments	+	+	−	+	+

T-PLL, T-cell prolymphocytic leukemia; T-LGL, T-cell large granular lymphocytic leukemia; ATLL, adult T-cell leukemia/lymphoma; MF/SS, mycosis fungoides/Sézary syndrome; sCD3, surface CD3; cCD3, cytoplasmic CD3; TCR, T-cell receptor.

+, positive; +/−, usually positive; −/+ usually negative; −, negative.

Aberrant loss of T-cell markers other than CD7 may also occur.

(Fig. 11.12). The classical morphologic type shows peripheral blood and bone marrow involvement by small to medium-sized lymphocytes with abundant cytoplasm and a prominent central nucleolus. The nuclei may be round to oval or may show slight nuclear convolutions. These cells cannot be reliably distinguished from B-cell prolymphocytes. A small-cell variant of T-PLL is also described (Matutes & Catovsky, 1996), and includes some cases that have been referred to historically as T-cell chronic lymphocytic leukemia, although use of this term is now discouraged. The tumor cells of this variant have less abundant cytoplasm, more condensed nuclear chromatin, and inconspicuous or absent nucleoli. This variant may present with a lower white blood cell count than the more usual type of T-PLL.

The neoplastic cells are usually CD4-positive with expression of surface CD2, CD3, CD5, and CD7, although aberrant loss of one or more T-cell antigens may be observed. CD8 or dual CD4/CD8 expression is less common. The cells do not express CD1 or TdT, helping

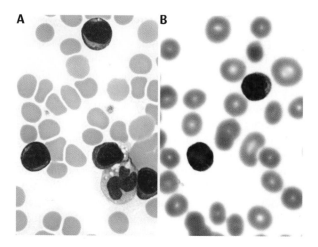

Figure 11.12. T-cell prolymphocytic leukemia (T-PLL). Some cases have features very similar to B-cell PLL (A), but many cases show smaller cells without a prominent nucleolus (B) and these are termed the small-cell variant of PLL.

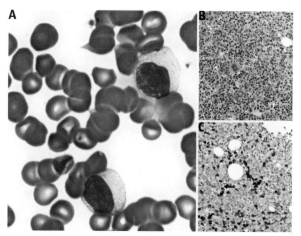

Figure 11.13. Large granular lymphocytic leukemia. (A) The peripheral blood shows large lymphocytes with abundant, granular cytoplasm. (B) The bone marrow changes are often subtle, but (C) aggregates of T cells that are CD3-positive are present. These clusters also express CD8 and granzyme B.

to exclude the possibility of T-cell acute lymphoblastic leukemia. T-cell receptor gene rearrangements are present and cytogenetic studies may reveal abnormalities involving the *TCL1* gene, including inv(14)(q11q32), t(14;14)(q11;q32), as well as trisomy 8 and abnormalities of the *ATM* gene at 11q22-q23 (Brito-Babapulle *et al.*, 1987b; Stoppa-Lyonnet *et al.*, 1998).

T-cell large granular lymphocytic leukemia and aggressive NK-cell leukemia

Large granular lymphocytic leukemia (Table 11.3) is a generally indolent chronic disease of T lymphocytes with prominent cytoplasmic granules that occurs in elderly patients (Loughran, 1993; Zambello & Semenzato, 1998). The patients often have a history of an autoimmune disease and may have mild splenomegaly, but no lymphadenopathy. T-cell large granular lymphocytic leukemia is associated with severe neutropenia and a prolonged elevation of large granular lymphocytes, usually above 2×10^9/L, for at least six months. Although bone marrow and splenic involvement are usually present, the diagnosis is primarily based on peripheral blood features and cell counts (Fig. 11.13). Bone marrow involvement is often subtle and interstitial on biopsy material, although an increase in large granular lymphocytes can usually be seen on aspirate smears. The lymphocytes are medium to large with abundant cytoplasm. They characteristically contain multiple azurophilic granules. The nuclei are round to oval with clumped nuclear chromatin without prominent nucleoli.

The cells are CD8-positive with expression of other T-cell-associated antigens, including surface CD3, as well as natural killer cell-associated markers CD16, CD56, CD57, TIA-1, and granzyme B. Interstitial clusters of CD8, TIA-1, or granzyme B-positive lymphocytes have been shown to be fairly specific for bone marrow involvement by T-cell large granular lymphocytic leukemia (Morice *et al.*, 2002). These proliferations are not associated with Epstein–Barr virus infection. T-cell receptor gene rearrangements are present. No recurring cytogenetic abnormalities are recognized.

Less commonly, cases with features similar to those described for T-cell large granular lymphocytic leukemia have a pure natural killer cell immunophenotype with no surface CD3 expression and absence of clonal T-cell receptor gene rearrangements. These cases may also express CD8. Some case of this type may represent indolent proliferations, including reactive NK-cell proliferations seen with viral infections. Cases with higher white blood cell counts, however, may represent true leukemias, including aggressive NK-cell leukemia (Sivakumaran & Richards, 1996; DiGiuseppe *et al.*, 1997) (Fig. 11.14). This disease may be more common in Asians and has systemic involvement with an aggressive clinical course. The cells express cytoplasmic but not surface CD3, and are CD56-positive. The neoplastic cells show cytoplasmic granules, but may have a more blastic nuclear appearance than most cases of T-cell large granular lymphocytic leukemia. The bone marrow may show subtle, or extensive and diffuse, involvement by disease. The possibility of a CD56-positive acute

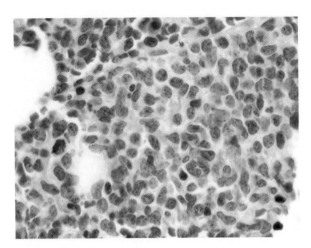

Figure 11.14. Blastic NK-cell leukemia. The bone marrow usually shows a diffuse infiltrate of intermediate-sized cells with a high mitotic rate and open chromatin that may suggest an acute myeloid leukemia.

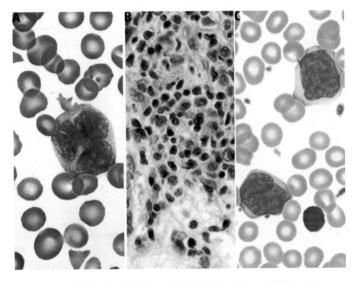

Figure 11.15. Adult T-cell leukemia/lymphoma (ATLL) and Sézary syndrome. (A) In adult T-cell leukemia the peripheral blood lymphocytes have convoluted nuclei. (B) The bone marrow in this case shows extensive fibrosis, with aggregates of lymphoma cells with irregular nuclei. (C) In Sézary syndrome the peripheral blood shows many large lymphocytes with irregular nuclei that have a cerebriform appearance.

myeloid leukemia should be excluded by demonstration of a lack of significant myeloid antigen expression and lack of cytochemical myeloperoxidase positivity. Aggressive NK-cell leukemia may be EBV-positive, and clonal cytogenetic abnormalities, including del(6)(q21q25), have been reported (Wong *et al.*, 1999).

Adult T-cell leukemia/lymphoma

Adult T-cell leukemia/lymphoma (ATLL) (Table 11.3) is a clonal T-cell proliferation, associated with HTLV-1 infection, that occurs most commonly in adults in the southeastern United States, Caribbean, west Africa, and southwest Japan (Jaffe *et al.*, 1984). It frequently presents with a leukemic phase, as well as lymphadenopathy, hepatosplenomegaly, and skin lesions. Hypercalcemia and lytic bone lesions are also common. The white blood cell count is markedly elevated due to the presence of abnormal lymphoid cells (Fig. 11.15). These cells are medium in size, usually with hyperlobulated "flower-like" or "knobby nuclei." Some cases may show less pleomorphic nuclear features (Tsukasaki *et al.*, 1999). The bone marrow is involved in just over half of cases, but it is usually normocellular. Despite the presence of extensive blood involvement, the marrow usually shows only focal or subtle involvement, with non-paratrabecular aggregates of atypical lymphoid cells (Jaffe *et al.*, 1984; Kikuchi *et al.*, 1992). Prominent osteoclastic activity and bone resorption are common in association with hypercalcemia.

The leukemic and bone marrow cells are CD4-positive T cells with expression of CD2, CD3, and CD5, but they are usually CD7-negative. Differing from most other chronic T-cell proliferations, the leukemic cells express CD25, and in contrast to T-lymphoblastic proliferations, the cells are TdT negative. Detection of T-cell receptor gene rearrangements and serologic or molecular evidence of HTLV-1 infection may be useful in confirming the diagnosis. Cytogenetic studies have reported the presence of multiple trisomies, 14q translocations, and 6q deletions in ATLL (Kamada *et al.*, 1992).

Mycosis fungoides/Sézary syndrome

Mycosis fungoides and its leukemic counterpart, Sézary syndrome (Table 11.3), are primarily cutaneous diseases that most often occur in adult males (Diamandidou *et al.*, 1996), but other organ involvement and focal bone marrow infiltration may occur. Peripheral blood Sézary cells may be small or large (Vonderheid *et al.*, 1985; Schechter *et al.*, 1987), although large cells should be present in the blood before a firm diagnosis is made, since small Sézary-like cells may be present in the blood with non-neoplastic skin lesions. The large diagnostic Sézary cell has scant to moderately abundant slightly basophilic cytoplasm. The nucleus is large with an irregular "cerebriform" appearance with nuclear clefts and dense or hyperchromatic nuclei (Fig. 11.15). Nucleoli are usually not prominent.

The bone marrow in mycosis fungoides and Sézary syndrome is usually normocellular, and even in the presence of extensive peripheral blood involvement may be only minimally involved or uninvolved (Salhany *et al.*, 1992; Graham *et al.*, 1993). An increase in marrow eosinophils may be present even in the absence of marrow disease. When marrow is involved, the lymphoid infiltration may be focal (nodular or interstitial), with aggregates of predominantly small cells with irregular nuclei. Admixed large, transformed cells may be present. Small aggregates may be difficult to distinguish from reactive lymphoid aggregates that are also usually predominantly T cells in the marrow.

The neoplastic cells are usually CD4-positive T cells and may show aberrant loss of one or more T-cell antigens. In contrast to ATLL, they are CD25-negative, and, in most cases, serologic or molecular evidence of HTLV-1 infection is not found. T-cell receptor gene rearrangement studies may be useful in confirming a suspicion of bone marrow involvement. Although cytogenetic abnormalities are common in mycosis fungoides and Sézary syndrome (Thangavelu *et al.*, 1997), no consistent recurring abnormalities have been identified.

Other peripheral T-cell lymphomas

Other types of T-cell lymphoma may involve the peripheral blood and bone marrow. As with most other aggressive lymphomas, they usually form distinct nodules in the bone marrow. They are frequently associated with focal marrow fibrosis and vascular proliferation, and may show admixed eosinophils and plasma cells (Fig. 11.16). These focal fibrotic lesions may raise a differential diagnosis with bone marrow involvement by Hodgkin lymphoma or mastocytosis, which also show fibrosis with associated eosinophils and plasma cells. The detection of CD30-positive Hodgkin cells, as described below, is necessary for a primary diagnosis of Hodgkin lymphoma in the marrow. Detection of aggregates of tryptase and CD117-positive mast cells in areas of fibrosis is helpful in making a diagnosis of mast cell disease (Yang *et al.*, 2000), which may be associated with other myeloproliferative or lymphoproliferative disorders.

Hodgkin lymphoma

Bone marrow involvement by classical Hodgkin lymphoma, including nodular sclerosis, mixed cellularity, lymphocyte-rich, and lymphocyte-depleted types, usually occurs in patients with a previous diagnosis of the disease. However, a primary diagnosis of Hodgkin lymphoma may

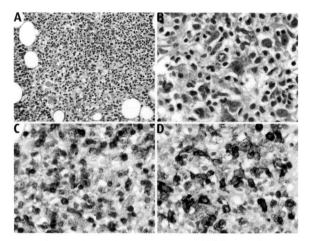

Figure 11.16. Angioimmunoblastic T-cell lymphoma. The bone marrow shows a nodular infiltrate (A) composed of a mixture of lymphocytes, plasma cells, and histiocytes (B). A CD3 stain highlights medium to large lymphocytes with irregular nuclear contours (C) and many of these cells also express CD10 (D), a feature typical of this disorder.

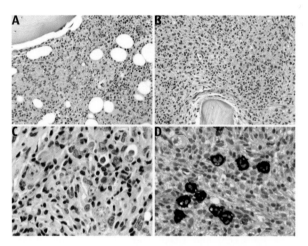

Figure 11.17. Classical Hodgkin lymphoma. The bone marrow may show histiocytic nodules (A) or a diffuse infiltrate (B) containing individual large pleomorphic cells with large eosinophilic nucleoli (C). These cells mark with CD30 (D) and CD15 (not shown), and are CD45-negative.

be made on bone marrow material. Although peripheral blood eosinophilia may occur with this disease, tumor cells are usually not seen in the blood. Disease involvement may be focal or diffuse, and is usually associated with fibrosis and a background of small lymphocytes, histiocytes, and eosinophils (Fig. 11.17). Bone marrow eosinophilia, lymphohistiocytic aggregates, and granulomas may occur in patients with nodal Hodgkin lymphoma, in the absence of true bone marrow involvement by disease, and these features should not be assumed to represent marrow disease (Kadin *et al.*, 1970). Therefore, Reed-Sternberg cells or their mononuclear variants must be identified in the marrow before a diagnosis of involvement by Hodgkin lymphoma is made. These cells are usually not evident on bone marrow aspirate smears, due to the associated marrow fibrosis, but may be seen on imprint preparations. The diagnostic cells are large with prominent eosinophilic nucleoli and may be multinucleated. They usually show a characteristic immunophenotype with expression of CD30 and PAX-5, variable positivity with CD15, but no expression of CD45, BOB.1, or OCT 2. A subset of the neoplastic cells may express CD20. In specimens that show lymphohistiocytic aggregates without large atypical cells, multiple tissue levels should be cut to exclude disease involvement.

The differential diagnosis of bone marrow involvement by classical Hodgkin lymphoma would include T-cell lymphomas and T-cell/histiocyte-rich large B-cell lymphoma. The expression of CD20 in some cases of classical Hodgkin lymphoma is usually only focal, and would be strong and diffuse in the large neoplastic cells of T-cell/histiocyte-rich large B-cell lymphoma. The lack of expression of CD45 in classical Hodgkin lymphoma is helpful in excluding bone marrow involvement by non-Hodgkin lymphoma of either B or T cell type. The neoplastic cells of Hodgkin lymphoma do not express CD43 or specific T-cell markers, which is also useful in the differential diagnosis of T-cell lymphoma.

Bone marrow involvement by nodular lymphocyte-predominant Hodgkin lymphoma is truly uncommon (Chang *et al.*, 1995), and cannot be reliably distinguished from T-cell/histiocyte-rich large B-cell lymphoma in the marrow. Large atypical cells with irregular or convoluted nuclear contours ("popcorn cells") are present, admixed with small lymphocytes. These cells are positive for CD20 and CD45 and do not express CD15 or CD30. Because the distinguishing features of nodular lymphocyte-predominant Hodgkin lymphoma and T-cell/histiocyte-rich large B-cell lymphoma require evaluation of the pattern of disease, definitive diagnosis of the lymphoma type would require examination of tissue other than the bone marrow.

Lymphoid aggregates

The presence of lymphoid aggregates in the bone marrow often creates diagnostic problems, especially when the bone marrow examination is performed to evaluate for possible lymphoma (Bluth *et al.*, 1993; Thiele *et al.*, 1999).

The frequent presence of discordant morphology between a diagnostic lymph node specimen and the cellular composition of the involved bone marrow forces the pathologist to regard all lymphoid aggregates of the marrow in patients with a known diagnosis of lymphoma with a high degree of suspicion (Robertson *et al.*, 1991). Reactive lymphoid aggregates are relatively common in elderly patients, as is malignant lymphoma. Reactive lymphoid aggregates may be identified on aspirate material, but are most commonly seen on clot or trephine biopsies. Reactive aggregates are usually well circumscribed, small, and non-paratrabecular in location. They are usually composed of predominantly small lymphocytes, but admixed medium and large lymphocytes, as well as histiocytes, are also common. Small intervening vessels are often associated with reactive lymphoid aggregates. Aggregates that are unusually large, paratrabecular in location, have irregular or infiltrating borders, or an atypical cell composition should be considered atypical and subjected to further evaluation.

Most reactive lymphoid aggregates are composed of predominantly CD3-positive T lymphocytes with smaller numbers of CD20-positive B cells, and the identification of this immunohistochemical pattern is useful in non-paratrabecular aggregates as long as there is not an increase in large B cells. Paratrabecular aggregates of follicular center cell lymphoma, however, often show a relatively high number of admixed reactive T lymphocytes, and a predominance of T cells with this pattern of infiltration should not be used to exclude involvement by lymphoma.

A predominance of B lymphocytes in an aggregate of any pattern is generally an indication of bone marrow involvement by B-cell lymphoma, with a few exceptions. With autoimmune disease, lymphoid aggregates with reactive germinal centers may be prominent, and these will show an increase in B cells (Farhi, 1989). The B cells, however, show a normal architectural pattern of the germinal center with surrounding small T lymphocytes, similar to what is seen in reactive germinal centers of lymph nodes. Reactive germinal centers may also rarely be seen in association with bone marrow involvement by certain lymphomas, particularly mantle cell lymphoma and marginal zone lymphoma. Increased numbers of small B cells in a diffuse pattern surround these aggregates, and this pattern should be considered as suspicious for lymphoma. Other clues to the diagnosis of marrow involvement by lymphomas of small B lymphocytes are aberrant co-expression of T-cell-associated markers CD43 and CD5, which most often occur with small lymphocytic lymphoma and mantle cell lymphoma. Flow cytometry immunophenotyping is often not useful in evaluating rare lymphoid aggregates, because the aggregates are often not present in the aspirate material submitted for these studies or too few cells are aspirated to detect an abnormal population.

In some cases, morphologically atypical lymphoid aggregates cannot be resolved by immunohistochemical study, and these should be considered indeterminate for involvement by malignant lymphoma (Cheson *et al.*, 1999). PCR analysis for *IgH* gene rearrangements of lymphoid aggregates microdissected from paraffin-embedded bone marrow biopsy may represent an additional technique for clonality assessment (Kremer *et al.*, 2000; Braunschweig *et al.*, 2003). The diagnostic value of this approach, however, has not yet been validated on an adequate number of cases.

REFERENCES

Arber, D. A. (2000). Molecular diagnostic approach to non-Hodgkin's lymphoma. *Journal of Molecular Diagnostics*, **2**, 178–90.

Bartlett, N. L. & Longo, D. L. (1999). T-small lymphocyte disorders. *Seminars in Hematology*, **36**, 164–70

Bennett, J. M., Catovsky, D., Daniel, M. T., *et al.* (1989). Proposals for the classification of chronic (mature) B and T lymphoid leukaemias. French–American–British (FAB) Cooperative Group. *Journal of Clinical Pathology*, **78**, 325–9.

Bluth, R. F., Casey, T. T., & McCurley, T. L. (1993). Differentiation of reactive from neoplastic small-cell lymphoid aggregates in paraffin-embedded marrow particle preparations using L-26 (CD20) and UCHL-1 (CD45RO) monoclonal antibodies. *American Journal of Clinical Pathology*, **99**, 150–6.

Bosch, F., Campo, E., Jares, P., *et al.* (1995). Increased expression of the PRAD-1/CCND1 gene in hairy cell leukaemia. *British Journal of Haematology*, **91**, 1025–30.

Braunschweig, R., Baur, A. S., Delacretaz, F., Bricod, C., & Benhattar, J. (2003). Contribution of IgH-PCR to the evaluation of B-cell lymphoma involvement in paraffin-embedded bone marrow biopsy specimens. *American Journal of Clinical Pathology*, **119**, 634–42.

Brito-Babapulle, V., Pittman, S., Melo, J. V., Pomfret, M., & Catovsky, D. (1987a). Cytogenetic studies on prolymphocytic leukemia. 1. B-cell prolymphocytic leukemia. *Hematologic Pathology*, **1**, 27–33.

Brito-Babapulle, V., Pomfret, M., Matutes, E., & Catovsky, D. (1987b). Cytogenetic studies on prolymphocytic leukemia. II. T-cell prolymphocytic leukemia. *Blood*, **70**, 926–31.

Catovsky, D., O'Brien, M., Melo, J. V., Wardle, J., & Brozovic, M. (1984). Hairy cell leukemia (HCL) variant: an intermediate disease between HCL and B prolymphocytic leukemia. *Seminars in Oncology*, **11**, 362–9.

Chang, K. L., Stroup, R., & Weiss, L. M. (1992). Hairy cell leukemia: current status. *American Journal of Clinical Pathology*, **97**, 719–38.

Chang, K. L., Kamel, O. W., Arber, D. A., Horyd, I. D., & Weiss, L. M. (1995). Pathologic features of nodular lymphocyte predominance Hodgkin's disease in extranodal sites. *American Journal of Surgical Pathology*, **19**, 1313–24.

Cheson, B. D., Bennett, J. M., Grever, M., *et al.* (1996). National Cancer Institute-sponsored working group guidelines for chronic lymphocytic leukemia: revised guidelines for diagnosis and treatment. *Blood*, **87**, 4990–7.

Cheson, B. D., Horning, S. J., Coiffier, B., *et al.* (1999). Report of an international workshop to standardize response criteria for non-Hodgkin's lymphomas. NCI Sponsored International Working Group. *Journal of Clinical Oncology*, **17**, 1244–53.

Chu, P. G., Chen, Y. Y., Molina, A., Arber, D. A., & Weiss, L. M. (2002). Recurrent B-cell neoplasms after Rituximab therapy: an immunophenotypic and genotypic study. *Leukemia and Lymphoma*, **43**, 2335–41.

Cohen, P. L., Kurtin, P. J., Donovan, K. A., & Hanson, C. A. (1998). Bone marrow and peripheral blood involvement in mantle cell lymphoma. *British Journal of Haematology*, **101**, 302–10.

Costes, V., Duchayne, E., Taib, J., *et al.* (2002). Intrasinusoidal bone marrow infiltration: a common growth pattern for different lymphoma subtypes. *British Journal of Haematology*, **119**, 916–22.

Crespo, M., Bosch, F., Villamor, N., *et al.* (2003). ZAP-70 expression as a surrogate for immunoglobulin-variable-region mutations in chronic lymphocytic leukemia. *New England Journal of Medicine*, **348**, 1764–75.

Damle, R. N., Wasil, T., Fais, F., *et al.* (1999). Ig V gene mutation status and CD38 expression as novel prognostic indicators in chronic lymphocytic leukemia. *Blood*, **94**, 1840–7.

Dayton, V. D., Arthur, D.C., Gajl-Peczalska, K. J., & Brunning, R. (1994). L3 acute lymphoblastic leukemia. Comparison with small noncleaved cell lymphoma involving the bone marrow. *American Journal of Clinical Pathology*, **101**, 130–9.

Diamandidou, E., Cohen, P. R., & Kurzrock, R. (1996). Mycosis fungoides and Sezary syndrome. *Blood*, **88**, 2385–409.

Diehl, L. F. & Ketchum, L. H. (1998). Autoimmune disease and chronic lymphocytic leukemia: autoimmune hemolytic anemia, pure red cell aplasia, and autoimmune thrombocytopenia. *Seminars in Oncology*, **25**, 80–97.

Dierlamm, J., Michaux, L., Wlodarska, I., *et al.* (1996). Trisomy 3 in marginal zone B-cell lymphoma: a study based on cytogenetic analysis and fluorescence in situ hybridization. *British Journal of Haematology*, **93**, 242–9.

Dierlamm, J., Baens, M., Wlodarska, I., *et al.* (1999). The apoptosis inhibitor gene *API2* and a novel 18q gene, *MLT*, are recurrently rearranged in the t(11;18)(q21;q21) associated with mucosa-associated lymphoid tissue lymphomas. *Blood*, **93**, 3601–9.

DiGiuseppe, J. A. & Borowitz, M. J. (1998). Clinical utility of flow cytometry in the chronic lymphoid leukemias. *Seminars in Oncology*, **25**, 6–10.

DiGiuseppe, J. A., Louie, D. C., Williams, J. E., *et al.* (1997). Blastic natural killer cell leukemia/lymphoma: a clinicopathologic study. *American Journal of Surgical Pathology*, **21**, 1223–30.

Dohner, H., Stilgenbauer, S., Dohner, K., Bentz, M., & Lichter, P. (1999). Chromosome aberrations in B-cell chronic lymphocytic leukemia: reassessment based on molecular cytogenetic analysis. *Journal of Molecular Medicine*, **77**, 266–81.

Espinet, B., Larriba, I., Salido, M., *et al.* (2002). Genetic characterization of the paraimmunoblastic variant of small lymphocytic lymphoma/chronic lymphocytic leukemia: a case report and review of the literature. *Human Pathology*, **33**, 1145–8.

Farhi, D. C. (1989). Germinal centers in the bone marrow. *Hematologic Pathology*, **3**, 133–6.

Ferry, J. A., Yang, W. I., Zukerberg, L. R., Wotherspoon, A. C., Arnold, A., & Harris, N. L. (1996). CD5+ extranodal marginal zone B-cell (MALT) lymphoma: a low grade neoplasm with a propensity for bone marrow involvement and relapse. *American Journal of Clinical Pathology*, **105**, 31–7.

Franco, V., Florena, A. M., & Campesi, G. (1996). Intrasinusoidal bone marrow infiltration: a possible hallmark of splenic lymphoma. *Histopathology*, **29**, 571–5.

Garand, R., Goasguen, J., Brizard, A., *et al.* (1998). Indolent course as a relatively frequent presentation in T-prolymphocytic leukaemia. Groupe Français d'Hématologie Cellulaire. *British Journal of Haematology*, **103**, 488–94.

Graham, S. J., Sharpe, R. W., Steinberg, S. M., Cotelingam, J. D., Sausville, E. A., & Foss, F. M. (1993). Prognostic implications of a bone marrow histopathologic classification system in mycosis fungoides and the Sézary syndrome. *Cancer*, **72**, 726–34.

Haglund, U., Juliusson, G., Stellan, B., & Gahrton, G. (1994). Hairy cell leukemia is characterized by clonal chromosome abnormalities clustered to specific regions. *Blood*, **83**, 2637–45.

Hamblin, T. J., Davis, Z., Gardiner, A., Oscier, D. G., & Stevenson, F. K. (1999). Unmutated Ig V(H) genes are associated with a more aggressive form of chronic lymphocytic leukemia. *Blood*, **94**, 1848–54.

Hoyer, J. D., Li, C. Y., Yam, L. T., Hanson, C. A., & Kurtin, P. J. (1997). Immunohistochemical demonstration of acid phosphatase isoenzyme 5 (tartrate-resistant) in paraffin sections of hairy cell leukemia and other hematologic disorders. *American Journal of Clinical Pathology*, **108**, 308–15.

Isaacson, P. G., Matutes, E., Burke, M., & Catovsky, D. (1994). The histopathology of splenic lymphoma with villous lymphocytes. *Blood*, **84**, 3828–34.

Jaffe, E. S., Blattner, W. A., Blayney, D. W., *et al.* (1984). The pathologic spectrum of adult T-cell leukemia/lymphoma in the United States: human T-cell leukemia/lymphoma virus-associated lymphoid malignancies. *American Journal of Surgical Pathology*, **8**, 263–75.

Jaffe, E. S., Harris, N. L., Stein, H., & Vardiman, J. W., eds. (2001). *World Health Organization Classification of Tumours: Pathology and Genetics of Tumours of Haematopoietic and Lymphoid Tissues.* Lyon: IARC Press.

Kadin, M. E., Donaldson, S. S., & Dorfman, R. F. (1970). Isolated granulomas in Hodgkin's disease. *New England Journal of Medicine*, **283**, 859–61.

Kamada, N., Sakurai, M., Miyamoto, K., *et al.* (1992). Chromosome abnormalities in adult T-cell leukemia/lymphoma: a karyotype review committee report. *Cancer Research*, **52**, 1481–93.

Kikuchi, M., Takeshita, M., Ohshima, K., & Yoshida, T. (1992). Pathology of adult T-cell leukemia/lymphoma and HTLV-1 associated organopathies. *Gann Monograph on Cancer Research*, **39**, 69–80.

Kremer, M., Cabras, A. D., Fend, F., *et al.* (2000). PCR analysis of IgH-gene rearrangements in small lymphoid infiltrates microdissected from sections of paraffin-embedded bone marrow biopsy specimens. *Human Pathology*, **31**, 847–53.

Lai, R., Weiss, L. M., Chang, K. L., & Arber, D. A. (1999). Frequency of CD43 expression in non-Hodgkin lymphoma. A survey of 742 cases and further characterization of rare CD43+ follicular lymphomas. *American Journal of Clinical Pathology*, **111**, 488–94.

Lambertenghi-Deliliers, G., Annaloro, C., Soligo, D., *et al.* (1992). Incidence and histological features of bone marrow involvement in malignant lymphomas. *Annals of Hematology*, **65**, 61–5.

Lens, D., Matutes, E., Catovsky, D., & Coignet, L. J. (2000). Frequent deletions at 11q23 and 13q14 in B cell prolymphocytic leukemia (B-PLL). *Leukemia*, **14**, 427–30.

Loughran, T. P. Jr. (1993). Clonal diseases of large granular lymphocytes. *Blood*, **82**, 1–14.

Matutes, E. & Catovsky, D. (1996). Similarities between T-cell chronic lymphocytic leukemia and the small-cell variant of T-prolymphocytic leukemia. *Blood*, **87**, 3520–1.

Matutes, E., Brito-Babapulle, V., Swansbury, J., *et al.* (1991). Clinical and laboratory features of 78 cases of T-prolymphocytic leukemia. *Blood*, **78**, 3269–74.

Matutes, E., Morilla, R., Owusu-Ankomah, K., Houliham, A., Meeus, P., & Catovsky, D. (1994). The immunophenotype of hairy cell leukemia (HCL): proposal for a scoring system to distinguish HCL from B-cell disorders with hairy or villous lymphocytes. *Leukemia and Lymphoma*, **14**, 57–61.

Matutes, E., Wotherspoon, A., & Catovsky, D. (2003). The variant form of hairy-cell leukaemia. *Best Practice and Research: Clinical Haematology*, **16**, 41–56.

Momose, H., Jaffe, E. S., Shin, S. S., Chen, Y. Y., & Weiss, L. M. (1992). Chronic lymphocytic leukemia/small lymphocytic lymphoma with Reed–Sternberg-like cells and possible transformation to Hodgkin's disease: mediation by Epstein–Barr virus. *American Journal of Surgical Pathology*, **16**, 859–67.

Morice, W. G., Kurtin, P. J., Tefferi, A., & Hanson, C. A. (2002). Distinct bone marrow findings in T-cell granular lymphocytic leukemia revealed by paraffin section immunoperoxidase stains for CD8, TIA-1, and granzyme B. *Blood*, **99**, 268–74.

Ott, G., Kalla, J., Hanke, A., *et al.* (1998). The cytomorphological spectrum of mantle cell lymphoma is reflected by distinct biological features. *Leukemia and Lymphoma*, **32**, 55–63.

Pangalis, G. A., Roussou, P. A., Kittas, C., *et al.* (1984). Patterns of bone marrow involvement in chronic lymphocytic leukemia and small lymphocytic (well differentiated) non-Hodgkin's lymphoma. Its clinical significance in relation to their differential diagnosis and prognosis. *Cancer*, **54**, 702–8.

Pettitt, A. R., Zuzel, M., & Cawley, J. C. (1999). Hairy-cell leukaemia: biology and management. *British Journal of Haematology*, **106**, 2–8.

Pritsch, O., Maloum, K., & Dighiero, G. (1998). Basic biology of autoimmune phenomena in chronic lymphocytic leukemia. *Seminars in Oncology*, **25**, 34–41.

Robertson, L. E., Redman, J. R., Butler, J. J., *et al.* (1991). Discordant bone marrow involvement in diffuse large-cell lymphoma: a distinct clinical–pathologic entity associated with a continuous risk of relapse. *Journal of Clinical Oncology*, **9**, 236–42.

Rozman, C., Montserrat, E., Rodriguez-Fernandez, J. M., *et al.* (1984). Bone marrow histologic pattern: the best single prognostic parameter in chronic lymphocytic leukemia. A multivariate survival analysis of 329 cases. *Blood*, **64**, 642–8.

Salhany, K. E., Greer, J. P., Cousar, J. B., & Collins, R. D. (1992). Marrow involvement in cutaneous T-cell lymphoma: a clinicopathologic study of 60 cases. *American Journal of Clinical Pathology*, **92**, 747–54.

Salomon-Nguyen, F., Valensi, F., Troussard, X., & Flandrin, G. (1996). The value of the monoclonal antibody, DBA44, in the diagnosis of B-lymphoid disorders. *Leukemia Research*, **20**, 909–13.

Schechter, G. P., Sausville, E. A., Fischmann, A. B., *et al.* (1987). Evaluation of circulating malignant cells provides prognostic information in cutaneous T cell lymphoma. *Blood*, **69**, 841–9.

Schlette, E., Bueso-Ramos, C., Giles, F., Glassman, A., Hayes, K., & Medeiros, L. J. (2001). Mature B-cell leukemias with more than 55% prolymphocytes: a heterogeneous group that includes an unusual variant of mantle cell lymphoma. *American Journal of Clinical Pathology*, **115**, 571–81.

Sivakumaran, M. & Richards, S. J. (1996). The clinical relevance of fluctuations in absolute-lymphocyte counts during follow-up of large granular lymphocyte proliferations. *Blood*, **88**, 1899–900.

Stilgenbauer, S., Bullinger, L., Lichter, P., Dohner, H., & German CLL Study Group. (2002). Genetics of chronic lymphocytic leukemia: genomic aberrations and V(H) gene mutation status in pathogenesis and clinical course. *Leukemia*, **16**, 993–1007.

Stoppa-Lyonnet, D., Soulier, J., Lauge, A., *et al.* (1998). Inactivation of the ATM gene in T-cell prolymphocytic leukemias. *Blood*, **91**, 3920–6.

Streubel, B., Simonitsch-Klupp, I., Müllauer, L., *et al.* (2004). Variable frequencies of MALT lymphoma-associated genetic aberrations in MALT lymphomas of different sites. *Leukemia*, **18**, 1722–6.

Taylor, A. M., Metcalfe, J. A., Thick, J., & Mak, Y. F. (1996). Leukemia and lymphoma in ataxia telangiectasia. *Blood*, **87**, 423–38.

Thangavelu, M., Finn, W. G., Yelavarthi, K. K., *et al.* (1997). Recurring structural chromosome abnormalities in peripheral blood lymphocytes of patients with mycosis fungoides/Sézary syndrome. *Blood*, **89**, 3371–7.

Thiele, J., Zirbes, T. K., Kvasnicka, H. M., & Fischer, R. (1999). Focal lymphoid aggregates (nodules) in bone marrow biopsies: differentiation between benign hyperplasia and malignant lymphoma. A practical guideline. *Journal of Clinical Pathology*, **52**, 294–300.

Torlakovic, E., Torlakovic, G., & Brunning, R. D. (2002). Follicular pattern of bone marrow involvement by follicular lymphoma. *American Journal of Clinical Pathology*, **118**, 780–6.

Tsukasaki, K., Imaizumi, Y., Tawara, M., *et al.* (1999). Diversity of leukaemic cell morphology in ATL correlates with prognostic factors, aberrant immunophenotype and defective HTLV-1 genotype. *British Journal of Haematology*, **105**, 369–75.

Vonderheid, E. C., Sobel, E. L., Nowell, P. C., Finan, J. B., Helfrich, M. K., & Whipple, D. S. (1985). Diagnostic and prognostic significance of Sézary cells in peripheral blood smears from patients with cutaneous T cell lymphoma. *Blood*, **66**, 358–66.

Wasman, J., Rosenthal, N. S., & Farhi, D.C. (1996). Mantle cell lymphoma: morphologic findings in bone marrow involvement. *American Journal of Clinical Pathology*, **106**, 196–200.

Wong, K. F., Zhang, Y. M., & Chan, J. K. (1999). Cytogenetic abnormalities in natural killer cell lymphoma/leukaemia: is there a consistent pattern? *Leukemia and Lymphoma*, **34**, 241–50.

Xu, Y., McKenna, R. W., & Kroft, S. H. (2002). Assessment of CD10 in the diagnosis of small B-cell lymphomas: a multiparameter flow cytometric study. *American Journal of Clinical Pathology*, **117**, 291–300.

Yang, F., Tran, T.-A., Carlson, J. A., His, E. D., Ross, C. W., & Arber, D. A. (2000). Paraffin section immunophenotype of cutaneous and extracutaneous mast cell disease: comparison to other hematopoietic neoplasms. *American Journal of Surgical Pathology*, **24**, 703–9.

Yegappan, S., Coupland, R., Arber, D. A., *et al.* (2001). Angiotropic lymphoma: an immunophenotypically and clinically heterogeneous lymphoma. *Modern Pathology*, **14**, 1147–56.

Zambello, R. & Semenzato, G. (1998). Large granular lymphocytosis. *Haematologica*, **83**, 936–42.

12

Immunosecretory disorders/plasma cell disorders and lymphoplasmacytic lymphoma

Introduction

Immunosecretory and plasma cell disorders cover a broad spectrum of clinical and pathologic entities. Some of the processes, such as monoclonal gammopathy of undetermined significance (MGUS), have relatively indolent behavior, while others, such as plasma cell leukemia, are associated with very poor prognosis and high mortality. This group of disorders includes lymphoplasmacytic lymphoma (LPL), a neoplastic entity which overlaps both with B-cell lymphoma and with the immunosecretory disorders group.

Benign plasma cells and reactive plasmacytosis

Plasma cells are a normal component of adult bone marrows. They typically represent about 0–1% of the overall cellularity seen in bone marrow aspirate smears (Foucar, 2001). Levels above 5% are considered abnormal in immunologically unstimulated marrows. In normal bone marrow biopsies, plasma cells are most typically located in perivascular locations.

In Wright–Giemsa-stained preparations, plasma cells have a distinctive, light to dark blue cytoplasm with an eccentrically placed nucleus. The nuclear chromatin is quite dense, and in appropriately thin histologic sections is classically described as "clockface chromatin." Adjacent to the nucleus is a clearing in the cytoplasm, referred to as a *hof*, which represents the Golgi apparatus of the cell.

The cytologic features of benign and malignant plasma cells can overlap (Fig. 12.1). Inclusions which may be seen in plasma cells include Russell bodies, which are globular eosinophilic collections of immunoglobulin in the cytoplasm. Dutcher bodies are not true nuclear inclusions but rather cytoplasmic inclusions that overlie the nucleus.

Dutcher bodies are only rarely seen in benign proliferations of plasma cells. Cells with multiple small globular cytoplasmic inclusions are termed Mott cells (or morula cells), the inclusions resembling bunches of grapes. Flame cells are a characteristic morphologic appearance seen in aspirate material, where the cytoplasm is centrally a typical deep blue color and the periphery of the plasma cell has a magenta or red color (Fig. 12.1). Flame cells can be seen in benign conditions, but when seen in myeloma, it is most often of IgA type. Very rarely, intracytoplasmic crystals or granules may be seen in plasma cells.

Reactive plasmacytosis is a relatively common finding in bone marrows (Gavarotti *et al.*, 1985). However, in the appropriate clinical context, reactive (polyclonal) plasmacytosis may have to be distinguished from the clonal expansion seen in cases of MGUS (see below for complete description of MGUS) or other plasma cell neoplasm. Benign plasmacytosis is usually characterized by cytologically mature-appearing plasma cells (Fig. 12.2). Immunoglobulin inclusions and other peculiar cytologic features can be seen in both benign and malignant plasma cells; however, their detection in more than occasional plasma cells may suggest a neoplastic rather than a benign proliferation.

Occasionally, in reactive conditions, the number of plasma cells (Gavarotti *et al.*, 1985; Nishimoto *et al.*, 1987; Poje *et al.*, 1992; Kass & Kapadia, 2001) may reach a frequency that would cause plasma cell myeloma to be considered in the differential diagnosis. In cases of viral hepatitis, especially hepatitis C, plasma cells can number up to 30–40% in the marrow. Chronic infections, autoimmune diseases, and hypersensitivity reactions can all cause varying degrees of polyclonal plasmacytosis. Chronic alcoholism may cause a mild plasmacytosis, typically not exceeding the 10% range. In addition, marrow involvement by plasma cell Castleman disease and in HIV/AIDS

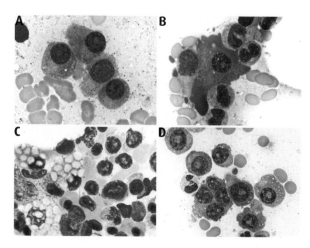

Figure 12.1. Cytologic feature of benign and neoplastic plasma cells. (A) Aspirate smear showing classic plasma cell morphology. (B) A flame cell, typically associated with IgA-secreting myeloma. (C) Plasma cells with multiple vacuoles of immunoglobulin (Mott cells). (D) Neoplastic plasma cells showing immature features including prominent single nucleoli, multinucleation, and centrally placed nuclei.

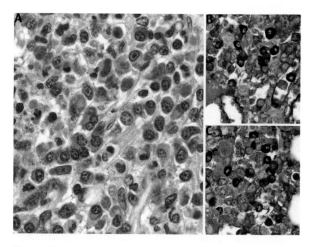

Figure 12.2. (A) Pronounced polyclonal plasmacytosis, in this case associated with hepatitis infection. Numerous plasma cells are present, including some atypical forms (e.g., binucleation and enlarged forms). (B) Kappa and (C) lambda immunohistochemical stains show a mixture of kappa- and lambda-staining plasma cells, confirming the polyclonal nature of the plasma cell proliferation.

may have striking marrow plasmacytosis. In HIV/AIDS, the plasma cells may have some morphologic features reminiscent of malignancy. These may be human herpes virus 8 (HHV-8) associated plasma cell proliferations, and may be precursors of HIV-related malignancies.

The most valuable distinction between benign plasmacytosis and neoplastic expansion is the presence, in the latter, of monoclonality by kappa/lambda light chain staining and/or the presence of a monoclonal serum and/or urinary immunoglobulin protein.

Monoclonal gammopathy of undetermined significance

Monoclonal gammopathy of undetermined significance (MGUS) refers to a clinical entity with production of a monoclonal protein without evidence of myeloma or other systemic lymphoproliferative disorder. The incidence increases with age, from about 1% at age 50 years to about 3% at age 70 years (Jaffe *et al.*, 2001; Kyle, 2003). Although most patients with this condition remain asymptomatic, approximately 25–30% go on to develop myeloma, amyloidosis, or more rarely other lymphoproliferative disorders (Kyle *et al.*, 2002; Kyle, 2003). As such, this entity can be considered as a precursor to other plasma cell neoplasms in some cases. The latency between discovery of MGUS and development of subsequent myeloma may be quite long, more than 10 years in some cases, so patients should be followed closely after a diagnosis of MGUS is made.

Because MGUS patients are asymptomatic, the monoclonal serum protein is usually discovered during a "routine" clinical evaluation inclusive of serum protein electrophoresis. The amount of serum monoclonal protein should be less than the criteria suggested for myeloma (IgG < 3.5 g/dL, IgA < 2 g/dL). The monoclonal protein is of IgG type in approximately 75% of cases. In addition, patients should lack any other symptoms of myeloma, and should not have radiologic evidence of skeletal lesions.

The bone marrow cellularity in MGUS has less than 10% plasma cells (Jaffe *et al.*, 2001). These plasma cells are virtually always morphologically mature. Immunohistologic evaluation for plasma cell clonality by kappa/lambda antibodies is frequently hampered by the small number of plasma cells, which is frequently insufficient for a reliable assessment of clonality. MGUS differs from indolent and smoldering myeloma based on the amount of serum monoclonal protein, the degree of plasmacytosis, and the presence of bone lesions (see below).

Plasma cell myeloma

Plasma cell myeloma (PCM), also referred to as multiple myeloma, accounts for approximately 15% of all

Table 12.1. Major and minor criteria for diagnosis of plasma cell myeloma (PCM).

Major criteria	Minor criteria
Bone marrow plasmacytosis >30%	Bone marrow plasmacytosis 10–30%
Plasmacytoma	Lytic bone lesions
Monoclonal protein Serum: IgG >3.5 g/dL, IgA >2 g/dL Urine: >1 g/24 hours of Bence–Jones protein	Monoclonal protein at levels less than those listed for major criteria
	Reduced normal immunoglobulins (<50% normal)

Adapted from Jaffe *et al.*, 2001. A diagnosis requires at least one major and one minor criterion, or three minor criteria which must include bone marrow plasmacytosis of 10–30% and a monoclonal protein of some level.

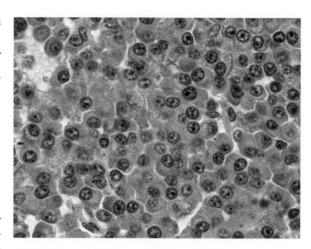

Figure 12.3. Bone marrow core biopsy showing extensive involvement with plasma cell myeloma (PCM).

hematopoietic neoplasms, and is the most common primary neoplasm of bone (Fletcher *et al.*, 2002). PCM is a rare disorder in persons less than 40 years of age, with incidence increasing with age. It is slightly more common in men than women, and is twice as common in blacks as in whites. Common signs and symptoms include bone pain, hypercalcemia, anemia, fatigue, renal failure, and recurrent infections.

Initial evaluation of patients with "overt" myeloma may be initiated because of symptoms, such as anemia or pathologic fracture. The diagnostic criteria for PCM are given in Table 12.1. In many cases, the total protein will be elevated, with a normal or low albumin, due to an increase in serum immunoglobulin. In other cases, the total protein may be normal, but with a significantly decreased albumin, with increased immunoglobulin protein accounting for the elevated total protein.

More than 95% of patients with PCM have abnormal serum or urine immunoglobulins. The monoclonal protein, or M-protein, can be of a variety of isotypes. The isotypes are present in the following proportions (Jaffe *et al.*, 2001):

IgG 55%
IgA 22%
light chain 18%
IgD 2%
IgE < 1%
IgM < 1%

These monoclonal proteins can be assessed in serum and urine by protein electrophoresis or by immunofixation.

Peripheral blood

In peripheral blood, PCM only occasionally has significant findings. Rouleaux is one of the more characteristic findings. Rouleaux is the formation of red blood cells into "stacks" of three cells or more, appearing like stacks of coins. This phenomenon is not exclusive to plasma cell dyscrasias and can be seen in reactive causes of hypergammaglobulinemia. In patients with PCM, the presence of rare circulating plasma cells can be occasionally seen. A significant number of circulating plasma cells is associated with a poor prognosis. Cases with numerous circulating plasma cells are more appropriately termed plasma cell leukemia (see below) (Jaffe *et al.*, 2001; Kyle, 2003).

Bone marrow

In most cases of PCM, the bone marrow cavities contain large aggregates or sheets of plasma cells; these cases do not usually represent a diagnostic challenge. One of the major criteria for diagnosing PCM (see Table 12.1) requires a frequency of marrow plasma cells of 30% (Fig. 12.3). Even in the presence of large numbers of plasma cells, proving light chain restriction is always necessary, either by serologic or by immunohistochemical studies. Lesser degrees of involvement (<30%) may still represent myeloma, if correlated with other clinical findings (skeletal survey, serum protein, etc.). Because of the patchy nature of involvement of PCM, there may be *bona fide* cases with 5% or less plasma cells in the sampled material. Similarly, dissociation between the plasma cell count obtained on bone marrow aspirate and biopsy is frequently seen. These circumstances should be taken in context of the complete evaluation of these patients.

Plasmacytic morphology is when the majority of the plasma cells present are mature. These have features of normal plasma cells with eccentric nuclei, condensed "clockface" chromatin, and a well-formed perinuclear *hof* in blue cytoplasm. Features of "immature" myeloma include any of the following: large nuclear size, nucleoli, centrally placed nuclei, and relatively open nuclear chromatin.

Cases with plasmablastic morphology (>2% plasmablasts) as defined on bone marrow aspirate smears (Greipp *et al.*, 1998; Rajkumar *et al.*, 1999) have a significantly worse prognosis. A plasmablast is defined as having a large nucleus, with open, reticulated (blastic) chromatin, a single large nucleolus, no or minimal *hof*, and deep blue cytoplasm. They may easily be mistaken for erythroid precursors. Unfortunately, plasmablasts are difficult to identify in bone marrow biopsies.

In many cases of myeloma, bone changes may be observed. These include the presence of bone trabeculae rimmed by prominent osteoblasts, and increased numbers of osteoclasts. In addition, thinned bone trabeculae are not uncommon. Rarely, there is osteosclerosis seen with myeloma. This may suggest a diagnosis of POEMS syndrome (see below).

Dysplastic features of other marrow elements may be often seen in patients with PCM. It is quite important to correlate dysplastic changes within the clinical context (e.g., recent chemotherapy) in order to avoid an erroneous interpretation of "clonal" myelodysplasia. True myelodysplastic syndromes may, however, be seen in association with PCM, both as a "*de novo*" condition or as a result of previous chemotherapy. Similarly, acute myeloid leukemias may develop in a patient with PCM or, rarely, may be concurrent with it.

Plasma cell myeloma variants

Indolent/smoldering myeloma
Indolent myeloma and smoldering myeloma are clinical variants of typical PCM. Indolent myeloma has serum protein levels that are diagnostic for myeloma, with 10–30% plasma cells in the marrow, but no other symptoms. Smoldering myeloma is similar but has lower limits on the levels of serum proteins allowable, only a limited number of bone lesions, and lacks other symptoms (Table 12.2).

Non-secretory
Rare cases of PCM (~1%) do not produce circulating immunoglobulin and are termed non-secretory myeloma. Because these patients do not have serologic evidence of

Table 12.2. Comparison of monoclonal gammopathy of undetermined significance (MGUS), indolent, and smoldering myeloma.

	MGUS	Indolent myeloma	Smoldering myeloma
Plasma cells in bone marrow	<10%	10–30%	>30%
Monoclonal protein	IgG <3.5, IgA <2	IgG >3.5, IgA >2	IgG 3.5–7, IgA 2–5
Lytic bone lesions	No	No	3 or fewer
Symptoms/infections	None	None	None

Adapted from Jaffe *et al.*, 2001.

M-protein, more emphasis is placed on the marrow findings. Monoclonality of plasma cells by immunohistochemistry or flow cytometry plays a more central role in this diagnosis. Rare cases of true "non-producing" myeloma have also has been reported. Clonality in these cases can only be established by molecular methods.

Plasma cell leukemia
Plasma cell leukemia (PCL) is a rare PCM variant with a predominant component of circulating plasma cells. It may present either *de novo* (primary PCL), or as a progression of pre-existing non-leukemic PCM (secondary PCL). It shares a similar dismal clinical outcome to PCM, but with a much accelerated course. The typical survival of patients with plasma cell leukemia is less than six months (Kyle, 2003).

The peripheral blood is characterized by circulating plasma cells of at least 2.0×10^9/L or >20% of the WBC. The morphology of the plasma cells varies from cytologically mature forms to plasmablasts, which can be morphologically indistinguishable from blasts of other types such as ALL or AML.

Anaplastic myeloma
Anaplastic myeloma is an aggressive variant of myeloma. Although a strict definition is lacking, it can be conceptualized as a myeloma that varies so much from the normal plasmacytic morphology that other neoplasms such as melanoma or carcinoma are considered in the differential diagnosis. These cases can have striking variation in size and shape, with irregular nuclei and only occasional features of normal plasma cells (Fig. 12.4). In these cases, a significant proportion of the neoplastic cells (>20%) should have anaplastic features. When strictly defined, anaplastic myeloma has a decidedly poor prognosis.

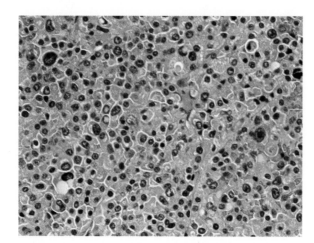

Figure 12.4. Anaplastic myeloma. Note that the atypical features of the cells are indistinct and could be confused with other lymphoproliferative disorders or metastatic malignancy.

Immunohistochemistry in plasma cell disorders

Immunohistochemical (IHC) analysis of bone marrow biopsy/clot sections can be of benefit in the evaluation of myeloma. Historically, IHC stains for immunoglobulin kappa and lambda light chains have been successfully used to demonstrate light chain restriction in plasma cells. Immunohistochemistry for light chains is sometimes difficult on decalcified bone marrow sections. For this reason, some laboratories now use *in situ* hybridization methods for detecting immunoglobulin light chains. Additional IHC stains that can be used to identify and quantitate plasma cells on core biopsy or clot section include CD38, CD138, and VS38c (Fig. 12.5). CD138 shows the most specificity for plasma cells and is frequently used. An important caveat is that CD138 can also be seen in a variety of non-hematopoietic cells and tumors, including melanoma (Chu *et al.*, 2003; O'Connell *et al.*, 2004). CD38 expression can be seen in a variety of proliferating lymphoid cells, particularly T cells, and is not specific for plasma cells. VS38c also lacks specificity, and staining may occasionally be seen in neuroendocrine tumors and melanoma.

CD56 may be useful in the evaluation of plasma cell proliferations. Approximately 70% of myeloma cases express CD56, whereas normal plasma cells do not. If positive, CD56 expression in plasma cells suggests malignancy. Additional stains may help distinguish neoplastic plasma cells from benign proliferations. Abnormal plasma cells may be positive for CD20 or CD10, which are only rarely expressed on a small minority of normal plasma cells. In addition, p53 and CD117 expression can be seen in malignant plasma cells. Positivity for these markers may be

Table 12.3. Immunohistochemical prognostic indicators in myeloma.

Stain	Prognosis
Cyclin D1	Good
p53	Poor
CD117	Poor
Increased proliferation (Ki-67)	Poor
CD56-negative	Poor

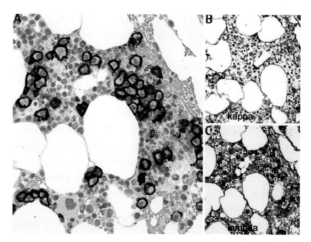

Figure 12.5. (A) CD138 stain highlighting plasma cells. (B) Kappa light chain stain showing no staining in the plasma cells. (C) Lambda light chain stain showing monoclonality.

associated with a poor prognosis in myeloma (Table 12.3). Cyclin D1 expression can be seen in a proportion of cases of myeloma. Positivity is restricted to the nucleus. In contrast to mantle cell lymphoma, only a small proportion of the neoplastic plasma cells are typically positive, even in myeloma cases with t(11;14). Most cases of PCM have a low proliferation rate. The presence of increased proliferation, as measured by either Ki-67 or DNA-S phase, is associated with a worse prognosis in PCM (Drach *et al.*, 1992).

Flow cytometry can play a significant role in the evaluation of PCM. Gating on the appropriate population (cells negative for CD45), plasma cells can be identified by markers such as CD138 (more specific) or CD38 (less specific). Since plasma cells do not express surface light chains, the cells must be made permeable to allow analysis of the cytoplasmic contents. This allows analysis of cytoplasmic light chains, from which monoclonality can be demonstrated. Flow cytometric analysis of plasma cell leukemia often differs for conventional PCM. Most notably, almost all cases of PCL are negative for CD56, an adhesion molecule that may be related to the bone marrow localization of PCM.

Cytogenetics in plasma cell disorders

Because of the limited mitotic index of plasma cells and most plasma cell neoplasms, cytogenetic analysis has historically been less utilized in plasma cell disorders. Using conventional cytogenetics, approximately 30% of myelomas show cytogenetic abnormalities. In addition, cases of recurrent or progressive disease have higher percentages of cytogenetic abnormalities. Fluorescence *in situ* hybridization (FISH) has been increasingly utilized in cytogenetic evaluation of myeloma and plasma cell disorders.

Two cytogenetic abnormalities are common in myeloma: deletions of 13q and translocations involving 14q32. Deletions of 13q and monosomy 13 are seen in up to 50% of cases of myeloma when analyzed by FISH (Drach *et al.*, 2000; Fonseca *et al.*, 2003). 13q14 is the most common site of deletion (e.g., retinoblastoma tumor suppressor gene), and it is associated with a poor prognosis.

Between 50% and 60% of patients with myeloma have translocations of the immunoglobulin heavy chain (IgH) with some other partner gene. These translocations may be an early step in myeloma pathogenesis, but they alone are not sufficient for neoplastic transformation. There are several translocation partners, but a few need specific mention. t(11;14)(q13;q32) causes a translocation of the IgH gene with the cyclin D1 gene, most commonly associated with mantle cell lymphoma. It is present in 15–20% of myeloma patients by FISH and appears to be associated with a relatively good prognosis in myeloma. Additional recurrent translocations are t(4;14)(p16;q32), associated with the fibroblast growth factor receptor 3, and t(14;16)(q32;q23), associated with overexpression of c-Maf. Both of these translocations are associated with a poor prognosis in myeloma. Besides these abnormalities are a variety of other cytogenetic abnormalities. p53 mutations (17p13) are not uncommon, particularly in relapsed or treatment-resistant disease, and are associated with a poor prognosis. Complex karyotypic abnormalities, monosomies, deletions, and trisomies can be seen in many cases, with variable impacts on prognosis.

Solitary plasmacytoma of bone and extraosseous plasmacytoma

Solitary plasmacytoma of bone consists of a single bone tumor composed of monoclonal plasma cells. There are no other sites of involvement in the bone marrow, skeleton,

or elsewhere. In addition, there are no other symptoms associated with myeloma. Approximately 30% of patients with solitary plasmacytoma of bone will go on to develop myeloma. Cases which occur in the base of skull seem to have a higher propensity to disseminate (Schwartz *et al.*, 2001).

Extraosseous plasmacytoma is a similar entity, but is located in tissues outside the bone. A common site is in the upper respiratory tract, including the sinonasal area. Extraosseous plasmacytoma has a relatively good prognosis, with only rare cases developing subsequent myeloma.

POEMS syndrome/osteosclerotic myeloma

Osteosclerotic myeloma is often a part of a very rare disease entity termed POEMS syndrome. POEMS syndrome, historically referred to as Crow–Fukase disease, classically displays the following features:

Polyneuropathy (due to demyelination)
Organomegaly
Endocrine disorders (diabetes, gynecomastia, testicular atrophy)
Monoclonal gammopathy
Skin changes (hyperpigmentation, hypertrichosis)

The patients with POEMS may have features overlapping with plasma cell-type Castleman disease. This includes an association with HIV/AIDS as well as with infection by HHV-8. There is typically only a small M-protein, which is almost always of lambda light chain (either IgG or IgA).

The bone marrow shows infiltration by monoclonal plasma cells, with features similar to those seen in typical myeloma, but only in relatively small numbers (typically less than 5%). In contrast to myeloma, instead of lytic lesions or prominent bone thinning, the bones are markedly thickened. Irregular cement lines can also be seen. Significant paratrabecular fibrosis can be seen, often with associated neoplastic plasma cells.

Amyloidosis

There are two main types of amyloid deposition disease: primary and secondary. Secondary amyloidosis, referred to as AA, is relatively common and involves the deposition of amyloid protein as an age-related phenomenon in many organs and tissues. There is no underlying disorder and this deposition is usually of little clinical significance.

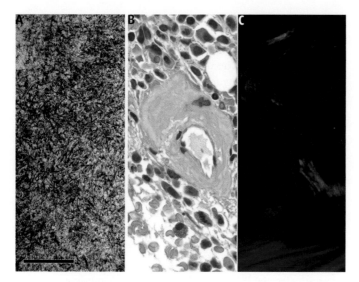

Figure 12.6. (A) An electron micrograph of amyloid showing the fibrillar nature of the protein. (B) Amyloid deposition in bone marrow. Note the glassy hyaline nature of the amyloid. (C) A Congo red stain of amyloid deposition with classic "apple-green" birefringence of amyloid in polarized light.

In contrast, primary amyloidosis (AL) is a disorder of deposition of monoclonal light chain protein (either kappa or lambda). As in other types of amyloidosis, the protein deposited is in a beta-pleated sheet form. They are composed of linear, non-branching fibrils with a tightly packed structure, giving amyloid many of its paracrystalline properties (Fig. 12.6). Underlying the deposition of the amyloid protein in AL is a neoplasm of monoclonal plasma cells. In primary amyloidosis, plasma cells are not seen in great numbers (Wolf *et al.*, 1986; Swan *et al.*, 2003) (Fig. 12.6). The marrow often contains amyloid, as well as other body sites including spleen, kidneys, lymph nodes, and soft tissues. Amyloid is often preferentially deposited in vessel walls. Later, it may become more diffuse and appear as amorphous sheets of pink material on H&E. The differential diagnosis of amyloid deposition is wide, when considering any pink amorphous material that may be deposited in the bone marrow. The classic evaluation of amyloid protein is accomplished through the Congo red stain. Congo red will stain deposited amyloid a brick-red color. Most characteristically, the stained material will show classic "apple green" color when polarized (Fig. 12.6). Other useful stains include Thioflavin T and sulfated Alcian blue. Immunohistochemical stains for light chains will often be non-contributory in the amyloid material (possibly due to the relatively inaccessible protein configuration), but may highlight the rare monoclonal plasma cells in the background.

It is important to remember that some low-grade B-cell lymphoproliferative disorders may be associated with amyloid deposition to varying degrees. The diagnosis of primary amyloidosis should be reserved for cases without evidence of other lymphoproliferative disease.

Monoclonal light and heavy chain deposition diseases

Light chain deposition disease differs from amyloidosis in several aspects. Although there is deposition of abnormal immunoglobulin light chain material, it (1) does not form beta-pleated sheets typical of amyloid and (2) does not stain with Congo red. The number of plasma cells seen in light chain disease is variable.

Heavy chain diseases are all exceedingly rare lymphoproliferative disorders that produce only immunoglobulin heavy chain, without significant light chain production. They are heterogeneous, and each type (gamma, mu, and alpha) has counterparts in other lymphoproliferative disorders. Gamma heavy chain disease (GHCD) has findings similar to lymphoplasmacytic lymphoma; mu heavy chain disease (MHCD) resembles CLL; alpha heavy chain disease is a variant of marginal zone lymphoma. Each has blood and bone marrow involvement similar to the disease mentioned. One notable difference occurs in MHCD: the presence of plasma cells with single, large cytoplasmic vacuoles. This finding is striking, but does not occur in all cases.

Lymphoplasmacytic lymphoma

Lymphoplasmacytic lymphoma (LPL) is an uncommon disorder characterized by a neoplastic proliferation of lymphocytes, plasma cells, and intermediate forms (plasmacytoid lymphocytes), most often with prominent bone marrow and peripheral blood involvement. Lymph nodal and splenic disease may also be present. The median age of presentation is 63 years and LPL is quite rare before the fifth decade. There is a slight male predominance (60% males). In virtually all cases, the serum monoclonal protein is of IgM isotype, although there are rare cases of IgA. The designation Waldenstrom macroglobulinemia (WM) has been used in the past for this disorder. LPL is the preferred terminology, while WM is restricted to a clinical syndrome associated with many cases of LPL. WM is characterized by symptoms of hyperviscosity in association with production of monoclonal IgM protein (or rarely IgA, as noted above). Symptomatology associated with the hyperviscosity may

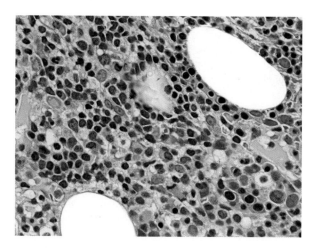

Figure 12.7. Lymphoplasmacytic lymphoma (LPL), showing multinodular marrow involvement with an atypical lymphoid infiltrate composed of a mixture of lymphocytes and plasma cells.

include neurologic symptoms, visual disturbances, and risk of cerebrovascular accidents.

Bone marrow

LPL may have a number of patterns of involvement in the bone marrow core, including interstitial aggregates, nodules, and diffuse (Fig. 12.7). Rarely, significant intrasinusoidal infiltration may be present. As in the peripheral blood, the neoplastic cells in the marrow consist of variable mixtures of small lymphocytes, plasmacytoid lymphocytes, and plasma cells. In the plasma cells, Dutcher bodies are quite common. As mentioned previously, these are nuclear pseudoinclusions of immunoglobulin protein. The Dutcher bodies can be highlighted by a PAS stain.

Ancillary studies

Immunohistochemical studies can be quite useful in delineation of LPL. Because there is often clear evidence of plasma cell differentiation, stains for immunoglobulin light chains can be of benefit in proving clonality. The neoplastic cells are typically positive for most pan-B-cell markers (CD20, CD79a, Pax-5). They are negative for CD5, CD10, and CD23.

Flow cytometry of LPL typically is positive for CD19, CD20, CD22, CD79a, HLA-DR, and plasma cell-associated antigens such as CD38 and CD138. LPL is negative for CD5, CD10, CD23, and IgD, which helps rule out other closely related entities.

Distinctions between lymphoplasmacytic and lymphoplasmacytoid types have been emphasized in the past. Distinguishing between these types has not been shown to be of clinical significance. LPL is a diagnosis of exclusion and should not be confused with other lymphomas of small lymphocytes with plasmacytoid features. With the increased recognition of marginal zone lymphoma involving the marrow, the number of cases of *bona fide* LPL has decreased significantly. In spite of this, LPL does represent a distinct clinical and pathologic entity. The differential diagnosis includes CLL/SLL with plasmacytoid features, marginal zone lymphoma, and other plasma cell disorders.

REFERENCES

Chu, P. G., Arber, D. A., & Weiss, L. M. (2003). Expression of T/NK cell and plasma cell antigens in non-hematopoietic epithelioid neoplasms: an immunohistochemical study of 447 cases. *American Journal of Clinical Pathology*, **120**, 64–70.

Drach, J., Gattringer, C., Glassl, H., Drach, D., & Huber, H. (1992). The biological and clinical significance of the KI-67 growth fraction in multiple myeloma. *Hematological Oncology*, **10**, 125–34.

Drach, J., Kaufmann, H., Urbauer, E., Schreiber, S., Ackermann, J., & Huber, H. (2000). The biology of multiple myeloma. *Journal of Cancer Research and Clinical Oncology*, **126**, 441–7.

Fletcher, C. D. M., Unni, K. K., & Mertens, F., eds. (2002). *World Health Organization Classification of Tumours: Pathology and Genetics of Tumours of Soft Tissue and Bone*. Lyon: IARC Press.

Fonseca, R., Blood, E., Rue, M., *et al.* (2003). Clinical and biologic implications of recurrent genomic aberrations in myeloma. *Blood*, **101**, 4569–75.

Foucar, K. (2001). *Bone Marrow Pathology*, 2nd edn. Chicago, IL: ASCP Press.

Gavarotti, P., Boccadoro, M., Redoglia, V., Golzio, F., & Pileri, A. (1985). Reactive plasmacytosis: case report and review of the literature. *Acta Haematologica*, **73**, 108–10.

Greipp, P. R., Leong, T., Bennett, J. M., *et al.* (1998). Plasmablastic morphology: an independent prognostic factor with clinical and laboratory correlates. Eastern Cooperative Oncology Group (ECOG) myeloma trial E9486. *Blood*, **7**, 2501–7.

Jaffe, E. S., Harris, N. L., Stein, H., & Vardiman, J. W., eds. (2001). *World Health Organization Classification of Tumours: Pathology and Genetics of Tumours of Haematopoietic and Lymphoid Tissues*. Lyon: IARC Press.

Kass, L. & Kapadia, I. H. (2001). Perivascular plasmacytosis: a light-microscopic and immunohistochemical study of 93 bone marrow biopsies. *Acta Haematologica*, **105**, 57–63.

Kyle, R. A. (2003). Plasma cell disorders. In *Atlas of Clinical Hematology*, ed. J. O. Armitage. Philadelphia, PA: Lippincott, Williams & Wilkins, pp. 119–36.

Kyle, R. A., Therneau, T. M., Rajkumar, S. V., *et al.* (2002). A long-term study of prognosis in monoclonal gammopathy of undetermined significance. *New England Journal of Medicine*, **346**, 564–9.

Nishimoto, Y., Iwahashi, T., Nishihara, T., *et al.* (1987). Hepatitis-associated aplastic anemia with systemic plasmacytosis. *Acta Pathologica Japonika*, **37**, 155–66.

O'Connell, F. P., Pinkus, J. L., & Pinkus, G. S. (2004). CD138 (syndecan-1), a plasma cell marker immunohistochemical profile in hematopoietic and nonhematopoietic neoplasms. *American Journal of Clinical Pathology*, **121**, 254–63.

Poje, E. J., Soori, G. S., & Weisenburger, D. D. (1992). Systemic polyclonal B-immunoblastic proliferation with marked peripheral blood and bone marrow plasmacytosis. *American Journal of Clinical Pathology*, **98**, 222–6.

Rajkumar, S. V., Fonseca, R., Lacy, M. Q., *et al.* (1999). Plasmablastic morphology is an independent predictor of poor survival after autologous stem-cell transplant for multiple myeloma. *Journal of Clinical Oncology*, **17**, 1551–7.

Schwartz, T. H., Rhiew, R., Isaacson, S. R., Orazi, A., & Bruce, J. N. (2001). Association between intracranial plasmacytoma and multiple myeloma: clinicopathological outcome study. *Neurosurgery*, **49**, 1039–45.

Swan, N., Skinner, M., & O'Hara, C. J. (2003). Bone marrow core biopsy specimens in AL (primary) amyloidosis: a morphologic and immunohistochemical study of 100 cases. *American Journal of Clinical Pathology*, **120**, 610–16.

Wolf, B. C., Kumar, A., Vera, J. C., & Neiman, R. S. (1986). Bone marrow morphology and immunology in systemic amyloidosis. *American Journal of Clinical Pathology*, **86**, 84–8.

13

Metastatic lesions

Introduction

Bone marrow biopsies performed to evaluate for metastatic disease are among the most common samples received. While advances in radiologic techniques have reduced the number of such bone marrow examinations, this method is still valuable for selected patients. Determination of the tumor type is usually not difficult in patients with a known primary tumor. However, unexpected malignancies may be identified, for example during an anemia work-up (Wong *et al.*, 1993), or bone marrow biopsy may be performed prior to a primary tumor biopsy. For example, a bone marrow biopsy may be performed as the initial procedure in a child with an abdominal mass. The ability to diagnose a tumor based on a bone marrow examination may reduce the need for further procedures or alter the approach of a second procedure. In the setting of an unknown primary, immunohistochemical studies are often essential for characterization. Even with these studies, clinical correlation is often needed to confirm the primary diagnosis. The most common non-hematologic malignancies to involve the bone marrow are prostate, breast, and lung carcinomas, neuroblastoma, Ewing sarcoma/peripheral neuroectodermal tumor (PNET), rhabdomyosarcoma, and malignant melanoma (Anner & Drewinki, 1977; Papac, 1994).

Peripheral blood and bone marrow aspirate

Peripheral blood involvement by metastatic tumor, termed carcinocythemia, is extremely uncommon and usually represents a late event with short survival (Gallivan & Lokich, 1984) (Fig. 13.1). Other, non-specific abnormalities of the blood are more common in patients with metastatic carcinoma. These usually manifest as anemia, leukoerythroblastosis, leukocytosis, and microangiopathic hemolytic anemia.

Tumor is often not easily identifiable on aspirate smears, but when present it is more often seen on the feathered edges of the smears as small clumps of cells (Fig. 13.2). The small round cell tumors of childhood, however, are relatively frequently detected on aspirate smears. Subclassification of these childhood tumors, however, is generally not possible on aspirate smears, and bone marrow biopsies are also advised when metastatic tumors are suspected (Delta & Pinkel, 1964). Aspirated tumor cells adequate for immunohistochemistry may be present on clot sections made from an aspirate, but clot sections alone may miss the presence of non-aspirated, focal disease that is best visualized on a core biopsy.

Bone marrow biopsy

The bone marrow trephine core biopsy is the most consistent means of detecting metastatic marrow disease. The optimal core biopsy length, and use of unilateral versus bilateral iliac crest biopsies, remain controversial. The optimal biopsy length for metastatic disease evaluation is not well defined, but lengths of at least 5 mm for pediatric specimens (Reid & Roald, 1996) and 10 mm for adult specimens have been used in the past. Areas of periosteum or cartilage, however, should not be included in the marrow length, and specimens containing very small amounts of marrow should be considered suboptimal for evaluation of metastatic disease. In addition, bilateral bone marrow biopsies are generally superior to unilateral biopsies for the detection of metastatic disease (Wang *et al.*, 2002). Some authors have suggested that two biopsies from the same iliac crest may be adequate for staging, although the sampling of bilateral sites appears to be superior to multiple

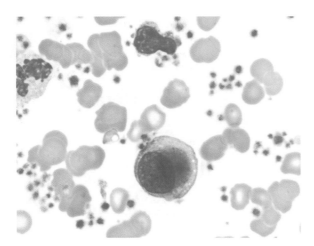

Figure 13.1. Peripheral blood involvement by breast carcinoma (carcinocythemia). This is a rare finding and often indicates a very poor prognosis.

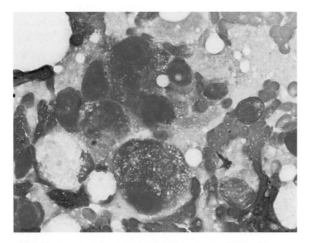

Figure 13.2. An aspirate smear showing a clump of malignant cells (malignant melanoma). Tumor clumps may be difficult to find. Sometimes, they are only seen at the periphery of the aspirate smear slide.

biopsies of a single site (Brunning *et al.*, 1975; Haddy *et al.*, 1989). The rate of tumor detection on bone marrow biopsy is also increased when more levels are examined (Jatoi *et al.*, 1999), and additional levels should always be obtained when suspicious foci are identified.

Metastatic tumors in adults

In adults, the majority of metastatic tumors are carcinomas or malignant melanoma, although sarcomas may

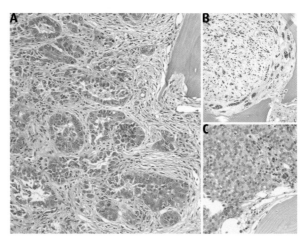

Figure 13.3. Metastatic neoplasms as seen in core biopsies. (A) Metastatic adenocarcinoma. (B) Metastatic lobular carcinoma of the breast. Early metastasis of this tumor may infiltrate as single cells in the marrow. (C) Metastatic adrenocortical carcinoma. Note the bland cytologic appearance. Pigmented material represents hemosiderin.

rarely involve the marrow. The routine use of immunohistochemical studies is usually not necessary in the evaluation of staging or in post-therapy marrows. Metastatic tumor cells are usually large, occur in aggregates, and have associated fibrosis with or without necrosis in the marrow (Fig. 13.3). When foci of fibrosis are present without obvious tumor, selected immunohistochemical studies may be useful to exclude tumor cells embedded within the fibrous stroma. Lobular carcinoma of the breast, however, often infiltrates the bone marrow as individual small cells without associated fibrosis and may be easily overlooked on H&E-stained sections alone (Bitter *et al.*, 1994; Lyda *et al.*, 2000). Because the detection of these individual cells within the marrow appears to have prognostic significance, routine staining of bone marrow biopsy and clot sections from patients with lobular carcinoma with a pan-keratin antibody is suggested. The identification of keratin-positive cells by immunohistochemistry allows for the re-review of the suspicious area on the routine section and usually identification of individual tumor cells on those sections.

Immunohistology can be helpful in confirming the origin of malignancy (Fig. 13.4). Immunohistochemical study for keratin, S-100 and CD45RB (leukocyte common antigen) are useful as part of an initial screen to identify keratin-positive carcinoma, keratin-negative, S-100-positive malignant melanoma, and large cell lymphoma (Table 13.1).

CD30 staining may be added if Hodgkin lymphoma is in the differential diagnosis. As indicated, additional

Table 13.1. Initial immunohistochemical panel for occult bone marrow large cell tumors in adults.

	Carcinoma	Melanoma	Lymphoma
Pan-keratin	$+^a$	−	−
S-100	−/+	+	−
CD45RB	−	−	$+^b$

^{a} Addition of keratin 7, keratin 20, chromogranin, TTF-1, estrogen receptor, and/or prostate-specific antigen may be useful for further classification.
^{b} The addition of lineage-specific lymphoid markers such as CD3 and CD20 is useful for further classification.

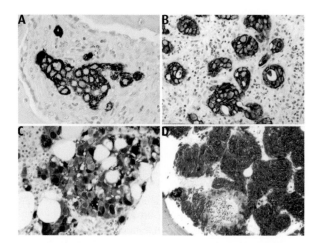

Figure 13.4. Metastatic neoplasms in core biopsies studied by immunoperoxidase staining. Immunohistology can be useful in determining the site of origin of a metastatic neoplasm.
(A) Keratin 7 (metastatic pancreatic adenocarcinoma). (B) Keratin 20 (metastatic colonic adenocarcinoma). (C) S-100 (metastatic melanoma). (D) NSE (small cell carcinoma of the lung).

immunohistochemical studies may be useful to identify estrogen receptor-positive breast or gynecologic carcinomas, prostate-specific antigen-positive prostate tumors, thyroid transcription factor-1 (TTF-1)-positive lung carcinomas, and chromogranin-positive small cell carcinomas. The more recent use of keratin-subset immunohistochemistry to identify metastatic tumors of unknown origin may also be applied to the bone marrow. Extensive surveys of keratin subsets in a wide variety of tumors have been reported (Wang *et al.*, 1995; Chu & Weiss, 2002; Chu *et al.*, 2002), with keratin 7 and keratin 20 staining being the most commonly used. Table 13.2 summarizes the profile of some of the more common metastatic carcinomas. It should be noted, however, exceptions to these patterns are

Table 13.2. Use of keratin subsets to evaluate metastatic tumors of unknown site.

Keratin profile	Tumor types
Keratin 7+/20+	Pancreatic carcinoma
	Transitional cell carcinoma
Keratin 7+/20−	Breast carcinoma
	Lung adenocarcinoma
	Ovarian adenocarcinoma
	Endometrial adenocarcinoma
	Thyroid carcinoma
	Mesothelioma
Keratin 7−/20+	Colonic adenocarcinoma
Keratin 7−/20−	Prostate adenocarcinoma
	Hepatocellular carcinoma
	Renal cell carcinoma
	Squamous cell carcinomas of multiple sites
	Adrenal cortical carcinoma
	Germ cell tumors

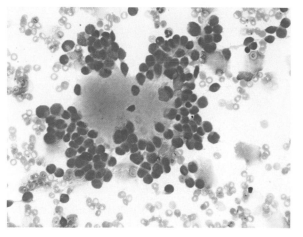

Figure 13.5. Aspirate smear of a "small blue-cell tumor" in a pediatric patient. The metastatic cells form a classic rosette in this case of neuroblastoma.

well reported and keratin subset staining should always be viewed in the context of the clinical setting.

Metastatic tumors in children

Pediatric sarcomas, particularly the small round cell tumors, frequently involve the bone marrow. While the tumor cells are frequently present on aspirate smears, showing clumps of large cells, distinguishing tumor types on smears is usually not possible (Fig. 13.5). The bone

Table 13.3. Use of immunohistochemical markers in differentiating among small round cell tumors of childhood.

	NB	ES/PNET	RMS	ML	ALL	AML
Vimentin	–	+	+	+	+/–	+/–
Pan-keratin	–	+/–	+/–	–	–	–
Desmin	–	–	+	–	–	–
CD99	–	+	–	+/–	+	+/–
Chromo/synapto	+	+/–	–	–	–	–
CD45RB	–	–	–	+	+/–	+
TdT	–	–	–	–	+	+/–
Myeloperoxidase	–	–	–	–	–	+

Chromo/synapto, chromogranin or synaptophysin; NB, neuroblastoma; ES/PNET, Ewing sarcoma/peripheral neuroectodermal tumor; RMS, rhabdomyosarcoma; ML, malignant lymphoma (mature); ALL, acute lymphoblastic leukemia/lymphoma; AML, acute myeloid leukemia.

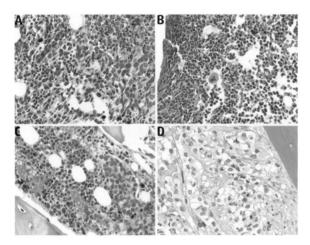

Figure 13.6. Core biopsy finding in pediatric marrows involved by metastatic tumors. (A, B) Metastatic neuroblastoma involving bone marrow. (C, D) Metastatic alveolar rhabdomyosarcomas involving bone marrow.

marrow biopsy may show clusters or sheets of tumor cells (Fig. 13.6). When present in sheets, these tumors may be confused with acute leukemias. The tumors display similar morphologic features and immunohistochemical staining profiles as seen in other sites, and a primary diagnosis can be made on a bone marrow biopsy specimen in many cases.

An initial immunohistochemical panel that includes vimentin, keratin, desmin, CD99, myeloperoxidase, and TdT is often helpful in the evaluation of these tumors (Askin & Perlman, 1998; Coffin & Dehner, 1998), and the staining patterns of the various tumors with these antibodies are listed in Table 13.3. Although CD99 is characteristic of Ewing sarcoma/PNET, acute lymphoblastic leukemia is also positive for this marker (Robertson *et al.*, 1997). TdT staining is helpful in this differential diagnosis and is positive in ALL while negative in Ewing/PNET. Additional staining for CD3 and CD79a will usually allow for further classification of TdT-positive ALLs.

REFERENCES

Anner, R. M. & Drewinki, B. (1977). Frequency and significance of bone marrow involvement by metastatic solid tumors. *Cancer*, **39**, 1337–44.

Askin, F. B. & Perlman, E. J. (1998). Neuroblastoma and peripheral neuroectodermal tumors. *American Journal of Clinical Pathology*, **109**, S23–30.

Bitter, M. A., Fiorito, D., Corkill, M. E., *et al.* (1994). Bone marrow involvement by lobular carcinoma of the breast cannot be identified reliably by routine histological examination alone. *Human Pathology*, **25**, 781–8.

Brunning, R. D., Bloomfield, C. D., McKenna, R. W., & Peterson, L. A. (1975). Bilateral trephine bone marrow biopsies in lymphoma and other neoplastic diseases. *Annals of Internal Medicine*, **82**, 365–6.

Chu, P., Wu, E., & Weiss, L. M. (2002). Cytokeratin 7 and cytokeratin 20 expression in epithelial neoplasms: a survey of 435 cases. *Modern Pathology*, **13**, 962–72.

Chu, P. G. & Weiss, L. M. (2002). Keratin expression in human tissues and neoplasms. *Histopathology*, **40**, 403–39.

Coffin, C. M. & Dehner, L. P. (1998). Pathologic evaluation of pediatric soft tissue tumors. *American Journal of Clinical Pathology*, **109**, S38–52.

Delta, B. G. & Pinkel, D. (1964). Bone marrow aspiration in children with malignant tumors. *Journal of Pediatrics*, **64**, 542–6.

Gallivan, M. V. & Lokich, J. J. (1984). Carcinocythemia (carcinoma cell leukemia): report of two cases with English literature review. *Cancer*, **53**, 1100–2.

Haddy, T. B., Parker, R. I., & Magrath, I. T. (1989). Bone marrow involvement in young patients with non-Hodgkin's lymphoma: the importance of multiple bone marrow samples for accurate staging. *Medical and Pediatric Oncology*, **17**, 418–23.

Jatoi, A., Dallal, G. E., & Nguyen, P. L. (1999). False-negative rates of tumor metastases in the histologic examination of bone marrow. *Modern Pathology*, **12**, 29–32.

Lyda, M. H., Tetef, M., Carter, N. H., Ikle, D., Weiss, L. M., & Arber, D. A. (2000). Keratin immunohistochemistry detects clinically significant metastases in bone marrow biopsy specimens in women with lobular breast carcinoma. *American Journal of Surgical Pathology*, **24**, 1593–9.

Papac, R. J. (1994). Bone marrow metastases: a review. *Cancer*, **74**, 2403–13.

Reid, M. M. & Roald, B. (1996). Adequacy of bone marrow trephine biopsy specimens in children. *Journal of Clinical Pathology*, **49**, 226–9.

Robertson, P. B., Neiman R. S., Worapongpaiboon, S., John, K., & Orazi, A. (1997). 013 (CD99) positivity in hematologic proliferations correlates with TdT positivity. *Modern Pathology*, **10**, 277–82.

Wang, J., Weiss, L. M., Chang, K. L., *et al.* (2002). Diagnostic utility of bilateral bone marrow examination: significance of morphologic and ancillary technique study in malignancy. *Cancer*, **94**, 1522–31.

Wang, N. P., Zee, S., Zarbo, R. J., Bacchi, C. E., & Gown, A. M. (1995). Coordinate expression of cytokeratins 7 and 20 defines unique subsets of carcinomas. *Applied Immunohistochemistry*, **3**, 99–107.

Wong, K. F., Chan, J. K., & Ma, S. K. (1993). Solid tumour with initial presentation in the bone marrow: a clinicopathologic study of 25 adult cases. *Hematological Oncology*, **11**, 35–42.

14

Post-therapy bone marrow changes

Introduction

A variety of therapy regimens and toxin exposures can cause bone marrow changes. Post-therapy evaluation of the marrow may be useful to evaluate for residual disease, to assess the degree of marrow ablation, or to look for signs of marrow recovery. While proper marrow evaluation after therapy in individual patients requires knowledge of the type of prior therapy and original disease, some changes after therapy are common to all cases and vary primarily by the degree of marrow ablation.

General marrow changes after myeloablative therapy

There are many similarities in the marrow findings following high-dose chemotherapy or combined chemotherapy and radiation, as is often used in preparation for hematopoietic stem cell transplantation, and even after toxin or drug injuries to the marrow (Sale & Buckner 1988; van den Berg *et al.*, 1989, 1990; Michelson *et al.*, 1993; Wilkins *et al.*, 1993). Common bone marrow changes after myeloablative therapy are summarized in Table 14.1. In the first week after the most severe types of injuries, the marrow shows complete aplasia with a complete or near-complete absence of normal hematopoietic elements and marrow fat. There is marked edema with dilated marrow sinuses, intramedullary hemorrhages, and scattered stromal cells, histiocytes, lymphocytes, and plasma cells. The histiocytes may contain cellular remnants, and fibrinoid necrosis may be prominent. Zonal areas of tumor necrosis may also be present, although myeloablative therapy is often given in the absence of prior marrow disease. After the first week, a mild reticulin fibrosis develops and the

reappearance of fat cells, often multilobulated, is the first evidence of marrow recovery (Fig. 14.1). Although the marrow remains markedly hypocellular, focal hematopoietic elements begin to appear in association with fat, usually in the second week after treatment. The regenerative islands may initially be composed only of erythroid cells or a mix of granulocyte precursors and erythroid cells, and both cell types can usually be identified after two weeks. By the third week, regenerating megakaryocytes, often hypolobated and in clusters, can usually be identified. Marrow regeneration in any age group, but most prominent in children, may also be associated with an increase in small lymphoid cells with a precursor B-cell immunophenotype, termed hematogones. These cells which show a spectrum of B-cell maturation are usually found admixed with other maturing marrow elements. As the marrow cellularity increases, the early reticulin fibrosis resolves and the marrow may become transiently hypercellular.

After recovery from hematopoietic stem cell transplantation, the marrow cellularity may remain patchy and below the pre-transplant cellularity, essentially establishing a new baseline cellularity for the post-transplant state (Fig. 14.2). Another unique general feature of the post-transplant marrow is a change in the maturation architecture of the marrow. While islands of regenerating marrow elements are normally located adjacent to bony trabeculae, the post-transplant marrow may show such islands away from bone, mimicking the so-called abnormal localization of immature cell precursors (ALIP) of myelodysplasia. Increases in siderotic iron are also common in post-transplantation states (Macon *et al.*, 1995), which may include the transient presence of ringed sideroblasts, and should not be interpreted as evidence of myelodysplasia.

Patients with delayed engraftment or post-therapy bone marrow failure show signs of aplasia for several weeks,

Table 14.1. Bone marrow changes in the three to four weeks following myeloablative therapy.

Initial changes
  Marrow aplasia
  Absence of fat cells
  Edema
  Fibrinoid necrosis with or without tumor necrosis
  Dilated sinuses
  Rare stromal cells, histiocytes, lymphocytes, and plasma cells
Intermediate changes
  Reappearance of fat, often lobulated
  Mild reticulin fibrosis
  Foci of left-shifted erythroid and granulocyte islands
  Increase in precursor B-cells on smears
Late changes
  Resolution of reticulin fibrosis
  Appearance of small megakaryocytes in clusters
  Normal or slightly increased marrow cellularity

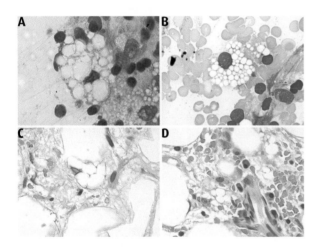

Figure 14.1. Early marrow changes after myeloablative therapy. Areas of multilobulated fat are common (A–D) as well as hypocellularity, with only scattered histiocytes, plasma cells, and lymphocytes present.

with histiocytes, stromal cells, lymphocytes, and plasma cells predominating (Rosenthal & Farhi, 1994). Delayed engraftment is more common in patients with marked marrow fibrosis prior to therapy (Soll *et al.*, 1995), and often shows a diffuse histiocytic proliferation of the marrow (Rosenthal & Farhi, 1994). Later marrow failure may occur secondary to viral infection, either primary or due to viral reactivation (Johnston *et al.*, 1999; Luppi *et al.*, 2000); and very late marrow failure may occur as a consequence of therapy-related myelodysplasia.

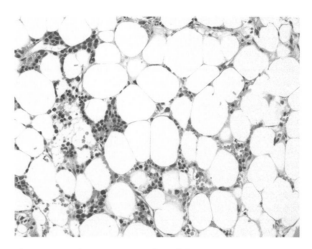

Figure 14.2. Characteristic patchy cellularity seen in a recovering post-transplant bone marrow.

Disease-specific changes after therapy

Some post-therapy bone marrow changes are somewhat disease- or therapy-specific. Evaluation of marrow residual disease by searching for tumor-specific immunophenotypic changes or molecular abnormalities has become more common and is reviewed in more detail elsewhere (Arber, in press). The use of novel therapies for some disease types, however, results in marrow changes that differ from those following combination chemotherapy. This section will focus on common diagnostic problems for specific disease types following therapy.

Acute leukemia

A bone marrow blast cell count of 5% is the traditional cutoff for the presence or absence of residual or recurrent leukemia, but this percentage is arbitrary and neoplastic clones can now be detected at much lower levels using multiparameter flow cytometry and molecular genetic methods (Xu *et al.*, 2002). These methods are beginning to redefine criteria for remission in acute leukemia. New criteria of response in acute myeloid leukemia define a "morphologic leukemia-free state" as less than 5% bone marrow blasts, with no Auer rods or extramedullary disease, as well as the absence of any aberrant leukemia immunophenotype by flow cytometry (Cheson *et al.*, 2003). A "morphologic complete remission" requires a morphologic leukemia-free state as well as an absolute neutrophil count of more than 1×10^9/L and a platelet count of more than 100×10^9/L. This definition no longer requires a minimum marrow

Table 14.2. Useful features in the differential diagnosis of hematogones and residual or recurrent precursor B-cell acute lymphoblastic leukemia.

Feature	Hematogones	Leukemia
Homogeneous nuclear chromatin	+	−
Maturation spectrum	+	−
Most cells smaller than a maturing granulocyte	+	−
Nucleoli	−	+
Precursor B-cell clusters on biopsy	−	+
Aberrant antigen expression	−	+/−
Peripheral blood involvement	−	+/−

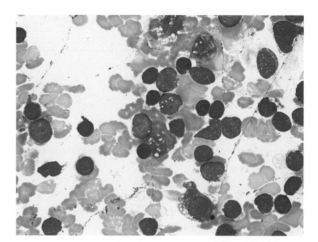

Figure 14.3. Residual acute lymphoblastic leukemia with post-treatment hematogone hyperplasia. Note the difference between the residual blasts (large, irregular nuclei, vacuolation) and the hematogones (small, dense mature chromatin, round nuclear contours). The distinction can be difficult, however, and flow cytometry or immunohistochemistry may be helpful.

cellularity for remission. The new criteria also have categories of "cytogenetic complete remission," "molecular complete remission," and "morphologic complete remission with incomplete blood count recovery." This later category is for patients that remain neutropenic or thrombocytopenic after chemotherapy.

Despite these new criteria, regenerative bone marrow blast cell increases of 5% or more may occur, especially with the common use of growth factors. Therefore, the simple use of a blast cell count is not sufficient for accurately determining the presence or absence of disease. Correlation with the original blast cell morphology and immunophenotype can be extremely helpful in this differential diagnosis.

A similar dilemma occurs in the differential diagnosis between residual or recurrent acute lymphoblastic leukemia and hematogones (Table 14.2). Hematogones are polytypic B-cell progenitors that usually show a spectrum of morphologic and immunophenotypic B-cell maturation, comparable to lymphoblasts (Fig. 14.3). In contrast to residual/recurrent leukemia, hematogones do not show aberrant antigen expression, usually do not involve the peripheral blood, and do not show prominent nucleoli. Therefore, the immunophenotypic detection of an aberrant leukemia clone or molecular testing for clonality may be useful in this differential diagnosis. Immunohistochemical study of the bone marrow biopsy may also be helpful in this setting. Detection of CD34- or TdT-positive immature cell clusters on the biopsy is helpful (Rimsza *et al.*, 1998), because regenerating blasts and hematogones do not normally form large clusters.

Acute promyelocytic leukemia

Most patients with acute promyelocytic leukemia receive both all-*trans*-retinoic acid (ATRA) and combination chemotherapy, and show post-therapy marrow changes

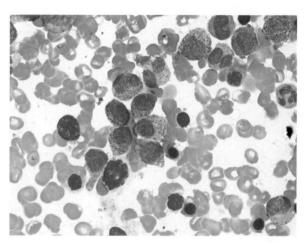

Figure 14.4. Post-therapy acute promyelocytic leukemia. Numerous residual promyelocytes are present, some of which are atypical in appearance.

that are similar to other acute myeloid leukemias. Some patients, however, are treated primarily with ATRA and do not develop post-therapy aplasia (Kantarjian *et al.*, 1985). The marrow may remain hypercellular, with elevated numbers of promyelocytes (Fig. 14.4). These cells will usually undergo a slow maturation secondary to the therapy. Therefore, the type of therapy should be known, as the presence of sheets of promyelocytes may not indicate treatment failure. These patients should be followed closely with additional marrow examinations and cytogenetic studies, to confirm that cell maturation is occurring and to confirm loss of the characteristic t(15;17) of this disease.

Chronic myelogenous leukemia

Busulfan, hydroxyurea, and α-interferon therapies have been commonly used to treat chronic myelogenous leukemia (CML), with some variation in the degree of bone marrow response. Some patients achieve clinical features of remission, with improvement of peripheral blood counts (Facchetti *et al.*, 1997; Thiele *et al.*, 2000). With busulfan, the bone marrow usually remains hypercellular with an elevated myeloid-to-erythroid ratio. Megakaryocytes tend to be increased with therapy, and this increase is associated with an increase in marrow fibrosis. With hydroxyurea, the marrow cellularity decreases somewhat, but usually remains above normal with only a moderate correction in the myeloid-to-erythroid ratio. The number of megakaryocytes and degree of marrow fibrosis, however, tend to decrease with hydroxyurea. With α-interferon, complete normalization of peripheral blood counts may occur. The bone marrow remains slightly hypercellular in most patients, but approximately one-quarter of patients will develop normal bone marrow features on α-interferon (Facchetti *et al.*, 1997). The number of marrow megakaryocytes remains elevated, with associated fibrosis, and bone marrow macrophages are also reportedly increased in these marrows. Despite the improvement in marrow cellularity, most patients continue to show cytogenetic evidence of clonal marrow disease.

Bone marrow transplantation is a standard treatment for CML in some centers (Snyder & McGlave, 1990). After transplantation, the marrow undergoes the expected changes of aplasia followed by regeneration. A majority of CML patients treated with transplantation are cured and will show normocellular or hypocellular marrows without specific abnormalities. Relapse specimens of patients treated with transplantation show changes similar to *de novo* disease, with granulocytic hyperplasia, basophilia, and hypercellularity, and are usually not diagnostic dilemmas.

Currently, many patients with all phases of CML are treated with imatinib mesylate, a tyrosine kinase inhibitor (Gleevec: Novartis, Hanover, NJ), that directly blocks the effects of the *BCR/ABL* fusion of t(9;22) (Kantarjian *et al.*, 2002). It results in a clinical, morphologic, and at least partial cytogenetic remission in many patients, with reduction in marrow cellularity, normalization of the myeloid-to-erythroid ratio, and normalization of megakaryocyte number and morphology (Braziel *et al.*, 2002; Hasserjian *et al.*, 2002). The peripheral blood is the first to respond

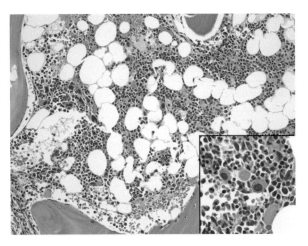

Figure 14.5. Post-imatinib therapy for chronic myelogenous leukemia. Note the decreased, normal-appearing cellularity. However, there are still residual stigmata of CML seen, including (*inset*) atypical, dwarf megakaryocytes.

to imatinib mesylate therapy, with a return to normal of the white blood cell count, decrease in basophils, and normalization of the platelet count, with normal-appearing platelets occurring after about two months of therapy. The hemoglobin level tends to decrease slightly during therapy. A subset of patients may develop neutropenia or thrombocytopenia while receiving the drug. The bone marrow hypercellularity gradually decreases and by 8–11 months the marrow is normocellular or hypocellular, with a normal or decreased myeloid-to-erythroid ratio in most patients. Bone marrow blast cells and megakaryocytes decrease, the number of hypolobated megakaryocytes decrease, and megakaryocyte clustering becomes less common as the marrow cellularity decreases (Fig. 14.5). This therapy has also been reported to gradually eliminate the marrow fibrosis that is prominent is some cases of CML (Beham-Schmid *et al.*, 2002; Braziel *et al.*, 2002; Hasserjian *et al.*, 2002). Patients with accelerated or blast phases of CML show similar changes, with rapid decreases in peripheral blood and bone marrow blast cell counts (Hasserjian *et al.*, 2002).

Because most therapies for CML result in near-normal cellularity and myeloid-to-erythroid ratios, it is often difficult to determine by morphologic features alone whether the disease is still present in the marrow. The most common clues to residual disease are hypercellularity, the presence of clusters of atypical megakaryocytes, and in some cases the continued presence of clusters of Gaucher-like histiocytes. Despite these clues, cytogenetic or molecular genetic studies for t(9;22) are needed to definitely determine the presence of continued involvement of disease.

Table 14.3. Changes associated with recombinant granulocyte colony-stimulating growth factor (G-CSF) and granulocyte–macrophage colony-stimulating growth factor (GM-CSF).

Peripheral blood changes
  Neutrophilia
  Granulocyte left shift
  Toxic granulation
  Dohle bodies
  Hypogranular neutrophils
  Vacuolated neutrophils
  Giant neutrophils
  Increase in large granular lymphocytes
  Eosinophilia
  Transient blast cells
  Circulating nucleated red blood cells
Early bone marrow changes
  Granulocytic hyperplasia with increase numbers
    of promyelocytes and myelocytes
  Transient blast cell increase
  Toxic granulation of granulocytes
  Enlarged promyelocytes and myelocytes
  Increased mitotic activity of granulocyte precursors
  Biopsy hypocellularity with left-shifted granulocytic precursors
Late bone marrow changes
  Binucleated promyelocytes
  Marrow neutrophilia
  Marrow eosinophilia
  Toxic granulation
  Variable biopsy cellularity

Growth factor changes

Growth factors are now administered for a variety of reasons, including enhancing bone marrow recovery after chemotherapy and priming the marrow or peripheral blood prior to stem cell collection (Armitage, 1998). It is essential that administration of these agents be included in the clinical history of any bone marrow sample. The most commonly administered growth factors are human recombinant granulocyte colony-stimulating factor (G-CSF) and granulocyte–macrophage colony-stimulating factor (GM-CSF). Both peripheral blood and bone marrow alterations occur with these drugs (Kerrigan *et al.*, 1989; Campbell *et al.*, 1992; Ryder *et al.*, 1992; Schmitz *et al.*, 1994; Meyerson *et al.*, 1998) (Table 14.3).

Both agents cause a peripheral blood leukocytosis with a granulocyte left shift. Toxic granulation and Dohle bodies are often present and may give the appearance of a reactive proliferation. Enlarged neutrophils or neutrophils with vac-

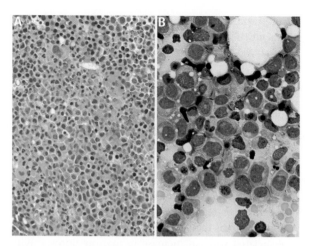

Figure 14.6. Colony-stimulating factor effects, after G-CSF administration. (A) Core biopsy shows a marked degree of neutrophilic hyperplasia. (B) Marrow aspirate smear displays the characteristic "maturation arrest" at the promyelocyte/early myelocyte stage which is seen during the early regenerative phase in patients with hypoplastic marrow treated with this cytokine.

uolated cytoplasm may also occur. The bone marrow shows a granulocytic hyperplasia which, depending on the timing of bone marrow examination, may display a complete spectrum of granulocytic maturation, may give the appearance of maturation arrest (Fig. 14.6), or may show a predominance of segmented neutrophils. The maturation arrest type changes that occur just after administration of the growth factor offer the most diagnostic problems and may be confused with recurrent leukemia or myelodysplasia. A predominance of promyelocytes and myelocytes is usually present. In rare cases, bone marrow and even peripheral blood blast cells may exceed 5% (Meyerson *et al.*, 1998), but this increase is usually accompanied by an increase in promyelocytes (Harris *et al.*, 1994). The transient increase in blast cells from growth factor administration should have even higher numbers of promyelocytes, and blast proliferations that are not accompanied by an increase in promyelocytes should be considered highly suspicious for leukemia and not simply attributed to growth factor changes.

In a patient with a history of acute myeloid leukemia, it may not be possible to entirely exclude the possibility of residual leukemia in the setting of an increase in blast cells, and cytogenetic studies or evaluation for a prior aberrant leukemia immunophenotype may be useful in that setting. The promyelocytes that occur with G-CSF and GM-CSF therapy usually have prominent perinuclear *hof*s, and this feature should be a clue to the possibility of growth factor administration. These cells differ from those of acute promyelocytic leukemia (Innes *et al.*, 1987); the latter usually do not show perinuclear cytoplasmic clearing, and demonstrate Auer rods that are not present in reactive promyelocytes. A repeat bone marrow examination one to two weeks after cessation of the growth factor will usually demonstrate more complete granulocyte maturation, and such a study is advisable in cases that are worrisome for residual leukemia. If true leukemic blast cells are present, they will persist or increase during this brief time interval, while reactive growth factor changes will resolve with time.

Less common changes that have been reported after G-CSF and GM-CSF therapy include marrow fibrosis (Orazi *et al.*, 1992), marrow necrosis (Katayama *et al.*, 1998), and marrow histiocyte proliferations (Wilson *et al.*, 1993), which may be confused with metastatic tumors (Pekarske & Shin, 1996).

Granulomas

The immunodeficiency associated with chemotherapy also increases these patients' risk for infectious diseases. Examination of the bone marrow is one means of evaluating patients for infections. If an infectious disease is suspected, fresh bone marrow aspirate material should be sent for microbiology studies. Histochemical stains for acid-fast and fungal organisms should be performed on all post-therapy biopsy specimens containing granulomas.

Necrosis

Bone marrow necrosis is a relatively uncommon finding, although the exact incidence is variable in the literature (Janssens *et al.*, 2000; Paydas *et al.*, 2002). When present, however, it is most commonly associated with marrow involvement by malignancy, and less frequently with infections, drug therapy, sickle cell disease, or other systemic abnormalities. The malignancies most often associated with marrow necrosis are acute leukemias, especially acute lymphoblastic leukemia, high-grade non-Hodgkin lymphomas, Hodgkin lymphoma, and metastatic carcinoma. Bone marrow necrosis may also be observed after chemotherapy. Bone marrow necrosis unrelated to anti-neoplastic therapy is discussed in Chapter 6.

Although not well studied, acute leukemias with marrow necrosis present prior to therapy appear to show post-therapy necrosis more commonly than specimens from patients that had non-necrotic pre-therapy specimens. Post-therapy necrosis usually shows complete marrow replacement by non-viable "ghost cells" with pyknotic nuclei and degenerative cytoplasm (Fig. 14.7). A careful

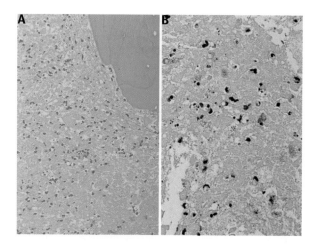

Figure 14.7. (A) Post-therapy necrosis. (B) Note the "ghosts" of blast cells in this case of acute myeloid leukemia.

examination should be performed to exclude the possibility of foci of viable residual tumor in these patients. Samples obtained in the course of or soon after therapy may entirely consist of large acellular areas of fibrinous, eosinophilic, necrotic material. Later, necrotic areas may be bordered by regenerating hematopoietic tissue. Areas of necrosis may be replaced by normal regenerating elements on follow-up specimens or may be replaced by fibrosis in subsequent biopsies. Post-therapy bone marrow necrosis caused by specific drugs is even less common, but has been reported with α-interferon, all-*trans*-retinoic acid, fludaribine, and G-CSF (Dreosti *et al.*, 1994; Katayama *et al.*, 1998; Janssens *et al.*, 2000).

Patients that have undergone prior therapy are also at high risk for infections, and infectious causes of marrow necrosis must also be considered in these patients. Special stains for organisms should be performed, especially when focal areas of necrosis are present in the marrow, even in the absence of granulomatous inflammation. If special stains are negative for organisms, repeat bone marrow aspiration for bacterial, fungal, or viral cultures should be considered if unsuspected necrotic foci are found that are not associated with necrotic tumor.

Fibrosis

Except for the development of fibrosis as part of the resolution of marrow necrosis, as mentioned previously, marrow fibrosis usually decreases or disappears after treatment of the primary disease by either chemotherapy or hematopoietic stem cell transplantation (Islam *et al.*, 1984). Development of marrow fibrosis after therapy may represent recurrence of disease or metastasis, or it may be secondary to non-neoplastic sequelae of the therapy. These secondary causes would be similar to the cause of marrow fibrosis in any marrow (McCarthy, 1985), such as fibrosis related to renal osteodystrophy, hypo- or hyperparathyroidism, or vitamin D deficiency. Patchy areas of fibrosis are also seen with bone marrow involvement by mast cell disease (Horny et al., 1985), which may accompany other hematologic malignancies at diagnosis or relapse (see Chapter 9).

REFERENCES

Arber, D. A. (2006). Evaluation of the post-therapy bone marrow. In *Diagnostic Hematopathology*, ed. E. S. Jaffe, N. L. Harris, & J. W. Vardiman. New York, NY: Harcourt.

Armitage, J. O. (1998). Emerging applications of recombinant human granulocyte–macrophage colony-stimulating factor. *Blood*, **92**, 4491–508.

Beham-Schmid, C., Apfelbeck, U., Sill, H., et al. (2002). Treatment of chronic myelogenous leukemia with the tyrosine kinase inhibitor STI571 results in marked regression of bone marrow fibrosis. *Blood*, **99**, 381–3.

Braziel, R. M., Launder, T. M., Druker, B. J., et al. (2002). Hematopathologic and cytogenetic findings in imatinib mesylate-treated chronic myelogenous leukemia patients: 14 months' experience. *Blood*, **100**, 435–41.

Campbell, L. J., Maher, D., W., Tay, D. L., et al. (1992). Marrow proliferation and the appearance of giant neutrophils in response to recombinant human granulocyte colony stimulating factor (rhG-CSF). *British Journal of Haematology*, **80**, 298–304.

Cheson, B. D., Bennett, J. M., Kopecky, K. J., et al. (2003). Revised recommendations of the International Working Group for diagnosis, standardization of response criteria, treatment outcomes, and reporting standards for therapeutic trials in acute myeloid leukemia. *Journal of Clinical Oncology*, **21**, 4642–9.

Dreosti, L. M., Bezwoda, W., & Gunter, K. (1994). Bone marrow necrosis following ALL-trans retinoic acid therapy for acute promyelocytic leukaemia. *Leukemia and Lymphoma*, **13**, 353–6.

Facchetti, F., Tironi, A., Marocolo, D., et al. (1997). Histopathological changes in bone marrow biopsies from patients with chronic myeloid leukaemia after treatment with recombinant alpha-interferon. *Histopathology*, **31**, 3–11.

Harris, A. C., Todd, W. M., Hackney, M. H., & Ben-Ezra, J. (1994). Bone marrow changes associated with recombinant granulocyte–macrophage and granulocyte colony-stimulating factors: discrimination of granulocytic regeneration. *Archives of Pathology and Laboratory Medicine*, **118**, 624–9.

Hasserjian, R. P., Boecklin, F., Parker, S., et al. (2002). STI571 (imatinib mesylate) reduces bone marrow cellularity and normalizes morphologic features irrespective of cytogenetic response. *American Journal of Clinical Pathology*, **117**, 360–7.

Horny, H. P., Parwaresch, M. R., & Lennert, K., (1985). Bone marrow findings in systemic mastocytosis. *Human Pathology*, **16**, 808–14.

Innes, D. J. Jr., Hess, C. E., Bertholf, M. F., & Wade, P. (1987). Promyelocyte morphology: differentiation of acute promyelocytic leukemia from benign myeloid proliferations. *American Journal of Clinical Pathology*, **88**, 725–9.

Islam, A., Catovsky, D., Goldman, J. M., & Galton, D. A. (1984). Bone marrow fibre content in acute myeloid leukaemia before and after treatment. *Journal of Clinical Pathology*, **37**, 1259–63.

Janssens, A. M., Offner, F. C., & Van Hove, W. Z. (2000). Bone marrow necrosis. *Cancer*, **88**, 1769–80.

Johnston, R. E., Geretti, A. M., Prentice, H. G., et al. (1999). HHV-6-related secondary graft failure following allogeneic bone marrow transplantation. *British Journal of Haematology*, **105**, 1041–3.

Kantarjian, H. M., Keating, M. J., McCredie, K. B., et al. (1985). A characteristic pattern of leukemic cell differentiation without cytoreduction during remission induction in acute promyelocytic leukemia. *Journal of Clinical Oncology*, **3**, 793–8.

Kantarjian, H., Sawyers, C., Hochhau, A., et al. (2002). Hematologic and cytogenetic responses to imatinib mesylate in chronic myelogenous leukemia. *New England Journal of Medicine*, **346**, 645–52.

Katayama, Y., Deguchi, S., Shinagawa, K., et al. (1998). Bone marrow necrosis in a patient with acute myeloblastic leukemia during administration of G-CSF and rapid hematologic recovery after allotransplantation of peripheral blood stem cells. *American Journal of Hematology*, **57**, 238–40.

Kerrigan, D. P., Castillo, A., Foucar, K., Townsend, K., & Neidhart, J. (1989). Peripheral blood morphologic changes after high-dose antineoplastic chemotherapy and recombinant human granulocyte colony-stimulating factor administration. *American Journal of Clinical Pathology*, **92**, 280–5.

Luppi, M., Barozzi, P., Schulz, T. F., et al. (2000). Bone marrow failure associated with human herpesvirus 8 infection after transplantation. *New England Journal of Medicine*, **343**, 1378–85.

Macon, W. R., Tham, K. T., Greer, J. P., & Wolff, S. N. (1995). Ringed sideroblasts: a frequent observation after bone marrow transplantation. *Modern Pathology*, **8**, 782–5.

McCarthy, D. M. (1985). Fibrosis of the bone marrow: content and causes. *British Journal of Haematology*, **59**, 1–7.

Meyerson, H. J., Farhi, D. C., & Rosenthal, N. S. (1998). Transient increase in blasts mimicking acute leukemia and progressing myelodysplasia in patients receiving growth factor. *American Journal of Clinical Pathology*, **109**, 675–81.

Michelson, J. D., Gornet, M., Codd, T., Torres, J., Lanighan, K., & Jones, R. (1993). Bone morphology after bone marrow transplantation for Hodgkin's and non-Hodgkin's lymphoma. *Experimental Hematology*, **21**, 475–82.

Orazi, A., Cattoretti, G., Schiro, R., et al. (1992). Recombinant human interleukin-3 and recombinant human granulocyte–macrophage colony-stimulating factor administered in vivo after high-dose cyclophosphamide cancer chemotherapy: effect on hematopoiesis and microenvironment in human bone marrow. *Blood*, **79**, 2610–19.

Paydas, S., Ergin, M., Baslamisli, F., *et al.* (2002) Bone marrow necrosis: clinicopathologic analysis of 20 cases and review of the literature. *American Journal of Hematology*, **70**, 300–5.

Pekarske, S. L. & Shin, S. S. (1996). Bone marrow changes induced by recombinant granulocyte colony-stimulating factor resembling metastatic carcinoma: distinction with cytochemical and immunohistochemical studies. *American Journal of Hematology*, **51**, 332–4.

Rimsza, L. M., Viswanatha, D. S., Winter, S. S., Leith, C. P., Frost, J. D., & Foucar, K. (1998). The presence of CD34+ cell clusters predicts impending relapse in children with acute lymphoblastic leukemia receiving maintenance chemotherapy. *American Journal of Clinical Pathology*, **110**, 313–20.

Rosenthal, N. S. & Farhi, D. C. (1994). Failure to engraft after bone marrow transplantation: bone marrow morphologic findings. *American Journal of Clinical Pathology*, **102**, 821–4.

Ryder, J. W., Lazarus, H. M., & Farhi, D. C. (1992). Bone marrow and blood findings after marrow transplantation and rhGM-CSF therapy. *American Journal of Clinical Pathology*, **97**, 631–7.

Sale, G. E. & Buckner, C. D. (1988). Pathology of bone marrow in transplant recipients. *Hematology/Oncology Clinics of North America*, **2**, 735–56.

Schmitz, L. L., McClure, J. S., Litz, C. E., *et al.* (1994). Morphologic and quantitative changes in blood and marrow cells following growth factor therapy. *American Journal of Clinical Pathology*, **101**, 67–75.

Snyder, D. S. & McGlave, P. B. (1990). Treatment of chronic myelogenous leukemia with bone marrow transplantation. *Hematology/Oncology Clinics of North America*, **4**, 535–57.

Soll, E., Massumoto, C., Clift, R. A., *et al.* (1995). Relevance of marrow fibrosis in bone marrow transplantation: a retrospective analysis of engraftment. *Blood*, **86**, 4667–73.

Thiele, J., Kvasnicka, H. M., Schmitt-Graeff, A., *et al.* (2000). Effects of chemotherapy (busulfan-hydroxyurea) and interferon-alfa on bone marrow morphologic features in chronic myelogenous leukemia: histochemical and morphometric study on sequential trephine biopsy specimens with special emphasis on dynamic features. *American Journal of Clinical Pathology*, **114**, 57–65.

van den Berg, H., Kluin, P. M., Zwaan, F. E., & Vossen, J. M. (1989). Histopathology of bone marrow reconstitution after allogeneic bone marrow transplantation. *Histopathology*, **15**, 363–73.

van den Berg, H., Kluin, P. M., & Vossen, J. M. (1990). Early reconstitution of haematopoiesis after allogeneic bone marrow transplantation: a prospective histopathological study of bone marrow biopsy specimens. *Journal of Clinical Pathology*, **43**, 365–9.

Wilkins, B. S., Bostanci, A. G., Ryan, M. F., & Jones, D. B. (1993). Haemopoietic regrowth after chemotherapy for acute leukaemia: an immunohistochemical study of bone marrow trephine biopsy specimens. *Journal of Clinical Pathology*, **46**, 915–21.

Wilson, P. A., Ayscue, L. H., Jones, G. R., & Bentley, S. A. (1993). Bone marrow histiocytic proliferation in association with colony-stimulating factor therapy. *America Journal of Clinical Pathology*, **99**, 311–13.

Xu, Y., McKenna, R. W., & Kroft, S. H. (2002). Assessment of CD10 in the diagnosis of small B-cell lymphomas: multiparameter flow cytometric study. *America Journal of Clinical Pathology*, **117**, 291–300.

Index